CLINICAL
SKILLBUILDERS™

Respiratory Support

D0057297

Springhouse Corporation
Springhouse, Pennsylvania

STAFF

Executive Director, Editorial
Stanley Loeb

Editorial Director
Matthew Cahill

Clinical Director
Barbara F. McVan, RN

Art Director
John Hubbard

Senior Editor
William J. Kelly

Clinical Project Editor
Joanne Patzek DaCunha, RN, BS

Editors
Barbara Delp, Margaret Eckman, Doris Falk, Kevin Law, Elizabeth Mauro

Clinical Editors
Patricia Holmes, RN, BSN; Sandra Ludwig Nettina, RN, MSN; Beverly Tscheschlog, RN

Copy Editors
Jane V. Cray (supervisor), Nancy Papsin, Doris Weinstock

Designers
Stephanie Peters (associate art director), Matie Patterson (senior designer), Julie Carlton Barlow, Linda Franklin

Illustrators
Dan Fione, Frank Grobelny, Robert Jackson, Robert Jones, Robert Neumann, Judy Newhouse, Larry Webb

Art Production
Robert Perry (manager), Anna Brindisi, Donald Knauss, Thomas Robbins, Robert Wieder

Typography
David Kosten (director), Diane Paluba (manager), Elizabeth Bergman, Joyce Rossi Biletz, Phyllis Marron, Robin Rantz, Valerie Rosenberger

Manufacturing
Deborah Meiris (manager), T.A. Landis, Jennifer Suter

Production Coordination
Colleen Hayman, Maura Murphy

Editorial Assistants
Maree DeRosa, Beverly Lane, Mary Madden

Library of Congress Cataloging-in-Publication Data
Respiratory support.
        p.   cm. – (Clinical skillbuilders)
        Includes bibliographical references and index.
        1. Respiratory organs – Diseases – Nursing.
2. Respiratory therapy.
I. Springhouse Corporation. II. Series.
        [DNLM: 1. Respiration, Artificial – handbooks.
2. Respiration, Artificial – nurses' instruction.
3. Ventilators, Mechanical – handbooks.
4. Ventilators, Mechanical – nurses' instruction.
WF 39 R4345]
RC735.5.R48   1991
615.8'36 – dc20
DNLM/DLC   90-10418
        ISBN 0-87434-362-3

CONTENTS

ADVISORY BOARD AND CONTRIBUTORS

At the time of publication, the advisors held the following positions.

Sandra G. Crandall, RN,C, MSN, CRNP
Director
Center for Nursing Excellence
Newtown, Pa.

Terry Matthew Foster, RN, BSN, CCRN, CEN
Clinical Director, Nursing Administration
Mercy Hospital-Anderson
Cincinnati
Staff Nurse, Emergency Department
St. Elizabeth Medical Center
Covington, Ky.

Sandra K. Goodnough-Hanneman, RN, PhD
Critical Care Nursing Consultant
Houston

Doris A. Millam, RN, MS, CRNI
I.V. Therapy Clinician
Holy Family Hospital
Des Plaines, Ill.

Deborah Panozzo Nelson, RN, MS, CCRN
Cardiovascular Clinical Specialist
Visiting Assistant Professor
EMS Nursing Education
Purdue University, Calumet Campus
Hammond, Ind.

Marilyn Sawyer Sommers, RN, MA, CCRN
Nurse Consultant
Instructor
College of Nursing and Health
University of Cincinnati

At the time of publication, the contributors held the following positions.

Karen Sudhoff Allard, RN, MSN, CCRN
Staff Development Educator, Critical Care
University of Cincinnati Hospital

Joanne Patzek DaCunha, RN, BS
Clinical Editor
Springhouse Corporation
Springhouse, Pa.

Sandra K. Goodnough-Hanneman, RN, PhD
Critical Care Nursing Consultant
Houston

Linda Foster Roy, RN, MSN, CCRN
Clinical Instructor, Critical Care
Doylestown Hospital
Doylestown, Pa.

Janet D'Agostino Taylor, RN, MSN
Pulmonary Clinical Specialist
St. Elizabeth's Hospital
Brighton, Mass.

FOREWORD

In recent years, two key changes have taken place in respiratory therapy. Thanks to improved diagnostic techniques, respiratory disorders are now detected in more patients than ever before. And because of increasingly sophisticated equipment, more types of treatment are available than ever before.

What do these trends mean for you? First, no matter where you work — in a hospital, a clinic, a long-term care facility, or in patients' homes — you can expect to provide respiratory support. Second, to give such support, you need not only a ready grasp of respiratory anatomy and physiology, but also a working knowledge of the vast array of respiratory equipment and techniques.

That's where *Respiratory Support,* part of the Clinical Skillbuilders™ series, will help. It gives you all the information you need in one handy, well-organized volume. The book explains in clear, common-sense language how the respiratory system works and how to perform essential respiratory procedures.

Respiratory Support begins by reviewing the underlying principles you need to know. The first chapter provides an in-depth discussion of respiratory anatomy and physiology — essential for understanding how respiratory disorders occur and how different treatments support diseased lungs.

Chapter 2 explains how to perform a respiratory assessment and focus on the findings that help in making effective treatment decisions. You'll learn how findings vary when a patient undergoes such treatments as mechanical ventilation. And you'll review how to perform the tests that

help you evaluate your patient's oxygen saturation, a crucial indicator of the success of respiratory support.

The next four chapters cover the types of respiratory support available, progressing from the least to the most invasive. Chapter 3 discusses airway maintenance. You'll find thorough explanations on how to perform chest physiotherapy as well as how to establish and maintain artificial airways. You'll also read about improved techniques, such as inflating an endotracheal cuff with minimal occlusive volume.

Chapter 4 reviews various ways of delivering oxygen from the simple nasal cannula to the Venturi mask. It explains how to set up the equipment you'll use and monitor the patient for complications.

Chapter 5 covers the types and modes of mechanical ventilation, as well as two adjuncts to therapy — continuous positive airway pressure and positive end-expiratory pressure. You'll read about how to set up and start a ventilator, provide patient care, prevent complications, prepare the family for home ventilator therapy, and wean the patient from a ventilator.

The final chapter explains chest drainage. Here you'll review how to assist with chest tube insertion, set up and monitor the drainage system, monitor your patient, and assist with chest tube removal.

Throughout the book, special graphic devices called logos call your attention to important aspects of respiratory therapy. The *Procedures* logo, for instance, signals a step-by-step explanation of a particular procedure, such as managing an airway obstruction. The *Equipment* logo indicates an in-depth look at a piece of equipment important for respiratory support—the Wright spirometer, for example. When you see the *Checklist* logo, you'll find important points to remember about a specific subject, such as caring for a ventilator patient receiving pancuronium. And the *Troubleshooting* logo catalogs measures you can take to quickly find and correct an equipment problem.

Following Chapter 6, you'll find a self-test, complete with answers at the end. This multiple-choice test lets you measure what you've learned and helps you further build your respiratory support skills.

With all this information, *Respiratory Support* is a valuable volume for any nurse who cares for respiratory patients. Whether you're a student, a recent graduate, or an experienced nurse, this book will serve as an indispensable resource. I recommend that you keep it handy so you can give your respiratory patients the excellent nursing care they deserve.

Gloria Sonnesso, RN, MSN, CCRN
Head Nurse, Medical Intensive Care Unit,
Intermediate Medical Unit,
and Controlled Environment Oncology Unit
Hahnemann University Hospital
Philadelphia

1

RESPIRATORY ANATOMY AND PHYSIOLOGY

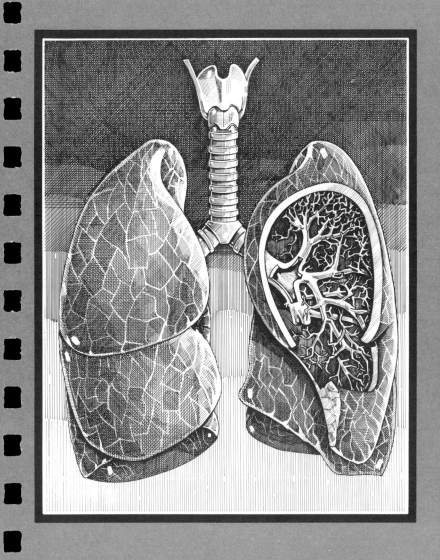

One in every five Americans suffers from some form of respiratory disease, ranging from chronic sinusitis to severe chronic obstructive pulmonary disease. Respiratory disease ranks as the second leading cause of disability and the sixth leading cause of death. What's more, the numbers are increasing, with mortality rising steadily by more than 1% each year.

In your practice, you'll care for patients who have severe chronic respiratory diseases as well as those who have residual respiratory impairment from a critical illness. You'll also care for patients who are living longer with their chronic conditions because of technological advances. These advances include direct measurements of alveolar oxygenation and carbon dioxide (CO_2) exchange, which more effectively monitor respiratory and metabolic status; ventilator refinements, which offer more flexibility in gas-flow delivery to compensate for specific pulmonary disorders; and improved tracheostomy and endotracheal tube design, which offers fewer complications and a higher survival rate for patients needing long-term management.

To meet the challenge of caring for these patients, you need to be proficient in the skills covered in this book. But before you focus on these skills, you should review the information that forms the basis of respiratory support—the anatomy, physiology, and pathophysiology of the respiratory system.

Anatomy

In one way or another, the respiratory system supports all vital functions. Besides its major function, exchanging CO_2 and oxygen (O_2), the respiratory system helps maintain the body's acid-base balance to ensure a stable hydrogen ion concentration. What's more, this system warms inhaled air, filters air through the nasal hairs, and distributes air through the vocal cords to allow speech.

Divided into upper and lower tracts, the respiratory system includes the organs and structures responsible for respiration. (See *Reviewing the respiratory system.*)

Upper respiratory tract
The upper respiratory tract consists of the nose, mouth, nasopharynx, oropharynx, larygnopharynx, and larynx.

Nose and mouth. During inspiration, air enters the body through the nostrils (nares), where small hairs (vibrissae) filter out dust and large particles. Separated by a septum, the two nasal passages are formed anteriorly by cartilaginous walls and posteriorly by light, spongy, bony structures known as conchae or turbinates.

Covered with a ciliated mucus layer, the conchae warm and humidify air before passing it through the nasopharynx. These tiny projections form eddies in the flowing air, forcing it to rebound in several different directions during its passage through the nose. This action traps finer particles, which the cilia then propel to the pharynx to be swallowed. If the air passage around the conchae is bypassed—for example, when a patient is on a ventilator—air must be humidified and heated outside the body.

The conchae also divide the nasal passages into the superior, middle, and inferior meatuses. The four

Reviewing the respiratory system

The illustration below shows the major structures of the respiratory system

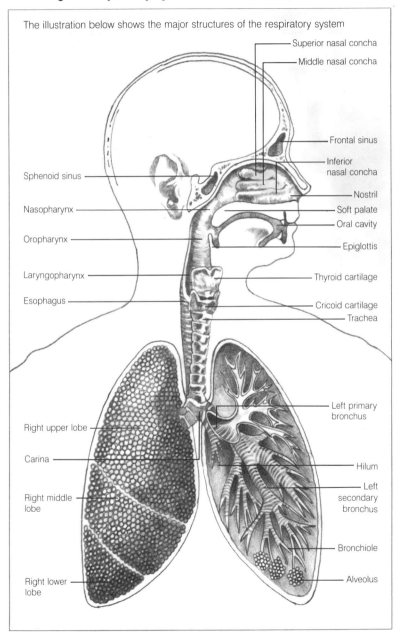

paranasal sinuses, which provide speech resonance, drain through these meatuses near the conchae.

The maxillary and frontal sinuses are large mucus-covered, air-filled cavities. The sphenoid and ethmoid sinuses — also mucus-coated — consist of several small spaces in the bony posterior portion of the nasal cavity.

Nasopharynx. Air flows from the nasal cavity through the conchae, which remain constantly open, into the muscular nasopharynx. The pharyngeal tonsils and the eustachian tube openings are nestled in the lateral walls of the nasopharynx above the soft palate. (The eustachian tubes regulate middle ear pressure.)

Oropharynx and laryngopharynx. The posterior wall of the mouth, the oropharynx, joins the nasopharynx to the laryngopharynx. Extending to the esophagus, the laryngopharynx is the lowest pharyngeal region.

Larynx. The larynx, which contains the vocal cords, connects the pharynx with the trachea by means of cartilaginous and muscular walls. Two of the trachea's nine cartilages — the thyroid cartilage (Adam's apple) and the cricoid cartilage just below the thyroid cartilage — can be palpated in the neck.

A leaf-shaped, flexible cartilage, the epiglottis hangs over the larynx. Its most important function is to prevent food or liquid from entering the airways. The epiglottis snaps shut during swallowing, routing food to the esophagus. It opens to allow air to enter and leave the trachea and lungs during inspiration and expiration.

The larynx aids coughing, an important protective mechanism. When dust, dirt, or other irritants

stimulate laryngeal sensory receptors, the abdominal and thoracic muscles contract against the diaphragm, increasing pressure in the tracheobronchial tree. The vocal cords open suddenly in a cough, forcing air and foreign particles out of the lungs.

Lower respiratory tract
The lower respiratory tract is subdivided into the conducting airways (trachea, primary bronchi, and secondary bronchi) and the acinus (respiratory bronchioles, alveolar ducts, and alveoli). The primary work of the respiratory system, gas exchange, takes place in the acinus. Mucous membrane lines the lower respiratory tract, and constant movement of mucus by ciliary action cleans the tract and carries foreign matter upward for swallowing or expectoration.

Trachea. The tubular trachea, half contained in the neck and half in the thorax, extends about 5″ (12 cm) from the only complete tracheal ring — the cricoid cartilage — to the carina at the level of the fifth thoracic vertebra. C-shaped cartilaginous rings reinforce and protect the trachea, preventing its collapse.

Bronchi. The trachea branches into two primary (mainstem) bronchi at the carina. The right primary bronchus, a more direct passageway from the trachea, is wider and about 1″ (2.5 cm) shorter than the left primary bronchus. As a result, aspirated particles entering the trachea — or a malpositioned endotracheal tube — are more likely to go into the right bronchus than the left. Like the trachea, the bronchi are reinforced with cartilaginous rings.

The primary bronchi divide into

five secondary (lobar) bronchi. Accompanied by blood vessels, nerves, and lymphatics, these bronchi enter the lungs at the hilum. Each secondary bronchus (right upper, middle, and lower, and left upper and lower) passes into its own lung lobe.

Bronchioles. Within its lobe, each secondary bronchus branches into smaller bronchi and finally into bronchioles. Each bronchiole, in turn, branches into lobules. The lobule includes the terminal bronchioles, which conclude the conducting airways, and the acinus, the chief respiratory unit for gas exchange. (See *Close-up look at a lobule.*)

Alveoli. Within the acinus, terminal bronchioles branch into respiratory bronchioles, which feed directly into alveoli at sites along their walls. These respiratory bronchioles end in alveolar sacs, clusters of capillary-swathed alveoli. Two-way gas diffusion occurs through the thin alveolar walls.

Alveoli consist of Type I and Type II epithelial cells. Thin, flat, squamous Type I cells, the most abundant, form the alveolar walls through which gas exchange occurs. Type II cells aid gas exchange by producing surfactant — a lipid-type substance that coats the alveolus, preventing total alveolar collapse, and facilitates gas exchange by decreasing surface tension.

Respiratory membrane. Alveolar cells, along with a minute interstitial space, capillary basement membrane, and endothelial cells in the capillary wall, collectively make up the respiratory membrane separating the alveolus and capillary. The entire structure normally is less

Close-up look at a lobule

As illustrated below, each lobule contains terminal bronchioles and the acinus, consisting of respiratory bronchioles and alveolar sacs.

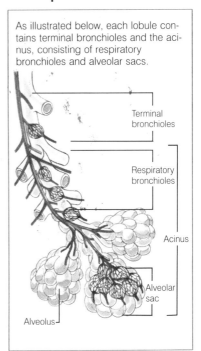

Terminal bronchioles

Respiratory bronchioles

Acinus

Alveolar sac

Alveolus

than 1 micron thick. Any increase in membrane thickness or decrease in surfactant production reduces the rate of gas diffusion across the membrane.

Lungs and accessory structures

Straddling the heart, the cone-shaped, spongy lungs fill the thoracic cavity, with the right lung shorter and broader than the left. Each lung's concave base rests on the diaphragm, and its apex extends slightly above the first rib. Lying above and behind the heart, the hilum provides an opening through which the primary bronchus, pulmonary and bronchial blood vessels, lymphatics, and nerves pass.

Except at the hilum, where ligaments anchor them, the lungs are freely movable. Along with the diaphragm, each lung base moves up during expiration and down during inspiration.

Fissures partially divide each lung into lobes — three lobes in the right lung and two in the left lung. The diaphragm, the floor of the thoracic cavity, separates the inferior surfaces of both lower lobes from the abdominal viscera.

Pleura. Composed of a visceral layer and a parietal layer, the pleura totally encloses the lung. A tough, elastic-like membrane, the visceral pleura hugs the contours of the lung surface, including the fissures between lobes, and separates each lung from mediastinal structures. The parietal pleura lines the inner surface of the chest wall, then doubles back around the mediastinum and meets the visceral pleura at the hilum to form a narrow fold known as the pulmonary ligament. Both the visceral and parietal pleurae contain connective and epithelial tissues and a single layer of secreting epithelium.

The airtight region between the pleural layers, the pleural cavity is only a potential space visible when air or fluid collects in it — as with pneumothorax or pleural effusion. Normally, a thin film of serous fluid fills this cavity, lubricating the pleural surfaces so they slide smoothly against each other and creating a vacuum between the layers, which compels the lungs to move synchronously with the chest wall during breathing.

Thoracic cavity. The area within the chest wall, the thoracic cavity is bounded below by the diaphragm, above by the scalene muscles and the fascia of the neck, and circumferentially by the ribs, intercostal muscles, vertebrae, sternum, and ligaments. The thoracic cavity houses vital organs and structures. The thoracic cage — the bones and muscles surrounding the thoracic cavity — protects the organs and supports the chest wall, allowing movement during respiration.

Mediastinum. Extending from the sternum to the vertebral column, the mediastinum consists of the space between the lungs. It houses the heart and pericardium, thoracic aorta, pulmonary arteries and veins, venae cavae, azygos veins, thymus, lymph nodes and vessels, trachea, esophagus, thoracic duct, and the vagus, cardiac, and phrenic nerves.

Pulmonary circulation

Blood being routed to the lungs for O_2 replenishment is pumped from the right ventricle to the pulmonary trunk. This trunk branches laterally into the right and left pulmonary arteries, which further divide into smaller arteries that follow the bronchial airways throughout the lungs. Eventually, these arteries branch into tiny arterioles. Together with minute branches of the pulmonary veins called venules, the arterioles form capillary beds and in the alveoli, the site of gas exchange. After O_2 diffusion occurs, oxygenated blood travels to the left atrium via the pulmonary veins. This blood is then pumped throughout the systemic circulation by way of the left ventricle.

Lung and pleural tissues receive blood from the bronchial arteries, which arise from the aorta and its branches. The bronchial arteries form part of the systemic circulation and play no part in the oxygenation of blood.

An extensive network of lymph vessels drains the pulmonary pleura in the dense connective tissues around the bronchi, respiratory bronchioles, pulmonary arteries, and veins. Circulating freely, lymph flows into collecting trunks, which empty into bronchopulmonary lymph nodes at the hilum.

Physiology

The respiratory system exchanges the CO_2 created by cellular metabolism for atmospheric O_2. Breathing, which produces this gas exchange, involves two actions: inspiration, an active process, and expiration, a relatively passive process. These two processes are regulated by neurologic and physical forces.

Neurologic control of breathing
A largely automatic and usually involuntary act, breathing is controlled neurologically by certain regulators and chemoreceptors and with the aid of certain physiologic factors (see *Innervation of respiratory structures*, page 8).

Neurologic regulators. Located in the medulla oblongata and the pons, respiratory centers actually are groups of scattered neurons that function as a unit to regulate breathing. At the primary location in the medulla—the medullary respiratory center—neurons associated with inspiration apparently interact with neurons associated with expiration to regulate respiratory rate and depth. These neurons react to impulses from other areas, particularly the pons.

In the pons, the apneustic center and the pneumotaxic center regulate respiratory rhythm. By interacting with the medullary respiratory center, these two neuron centers of the pons smooth the transitions from inspiration to expiration and back. The apneustic center of the pons stimulates inspiratory neurons in the medulla to trigger inspiration. In turn, these inspiratory neurons stimulate the pneumotaxic center of the pons to trigger expiration. They do this in two ways: by inhibiting the apneustic center and by stimulating the expiratory neurons in the medulla. Thus, the pons, as pacemaker, regulates rhythm, and the medulla regulates rate and depth.

Conscious control of breathing through nerve impulses from the motor areas of the cerebral cortex can override the involuntary respiratory centers. This permits voluntary breath control for such activities as speaking, singing, and swimming. But this conscious control can be exerted only temporarily. Eventually, the respiratory centers override the cortical impulses to meet ventilatory needs.

Central and peripheral chemoreceptors. Responding to changes in blood CO_2, O_2, and pH, these chemoreceptors monitor the body's ventilatory status and signal the respiratory centers to adjust respiratory rate and depth. The central chemoreceptors, located in the anterior medulla, are particularly sensitive to changes in partial pressure of carbon dioxide (PCO_2) and acid-base balance.

Here's an example of how these central chemoreceptors work. Physical exertion raises the level of CO_2 in the blood, and the gas diffuses easily from the cerebral capillaries into the cerebrospinal fluid bathing the central nervous system (CNS). Then the CO_2 reacts with water

Innervation of respiratory structures

Higher brain centers as well as other sources stimulate the respiratory centers in the pons and medulla. These centers then send impulses to various respiratory structures, altering respiratory patterns.

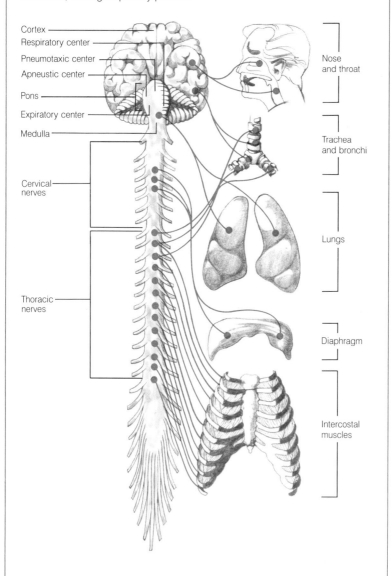

Cortex
Respiratory center
Pneumotaxic center
Apneustic center
Pons
Expiratory center
Medulla
Cervical nerves
Thoracic nerves

Nose and throat
Trachea and bronchi
Lungs
Diaphragm
Intercostal muscles

to form carbonic acid and yield hydrogen ions. The chemoreceptors detect this rising acidity and stimulate the respiratory centers to increase the respiratory rate and depth. As expiration of CO_2 lowers carbonic acid levels, the chemoreceptors stimulate the respiratory centers to decrease the respiratory rate and depth. Conversely, if blood levels of CO_2 drop below normal, the central chemoreceptors cause apnea until ongoing cellular metabolism produces enough CO_2 to stimulate the respiratory centers again.

Peripheral chemoreceptors, located in the aortic and carotid bodies, primarily monitor the blood O_2 level. When it falls, the O_2 content of interstitial fluid around the peripheral chemoreceptors falls too. In response, these receptors stimulate the respiratory centers to increase the respiratory rate or depth.

Physiologic factors. Several physiologic factors also significantly affect the neurologic control of breathing. These include lung inflation, changes in blood pressure and temperature, airway irritation, and sensory stimulation.

• *Lung inflation.* This action stimulates stretch receptors in the alveolar ducts, which send impulses along the vagus nerve to the CNS. These afferent impulses inhibit the inspiratory center, which then stops sending expansion impulses to the diaphragm and external intercostal muscles. Thus, these muscles stop expanding, and passive expiration follows.

This reflex — called the Hering-Breuer reflex — provides an important regulator of normal respiration. But another mechanism regulates respiration when the Hering-Breuer reflex is blocked. If the vagus nerve is cut, inspiration will be prolonged and deepened, but eventually the inspiratory center will stop sending expansion messages and allow expiration to occur.

• *Blood pressure changes.* Sudden, sharp changes stimulate pressoreceptors in the aortic and carotid sinuses. With a sudden rise in blood pressure, the receptors send impulses along the vagus and glossopharyngeal nerves to the respiratory centers. These impulses depress respiratory activity, temporarily making respirations slower and shallower. With a sudden blood pressure drop, as occurs with severe hemorrhage, pressoreceptor impulses slow, and respiratory center activity quickens correspondingly, increasing respiratory rate and depth.

• *Temperature changes.* Changes in the temperature of the blood passing through the respiratory centers can trigger changes in respiration. A temperature increase during fever or exertion quickens the respiratory rate; a temperature drop, as in hypothermia, slows the respiratory rate.

• *Airway irritation.* Foreign particles stimulate the protective "irritant" receptors in the mucous membrane that lines the respiratory tract. In the nose, this causes a sneeze to expel the irritant. In the larynx or trachea, such invasion induces a cough.

• *Sensory stimulation.* Stimulation of various receptors may cause a temporary reflex reaction. Sudden heat or cold exposure or alarming sights or sounds may provoke a gasp, an accelerated respiratory rate, or momentary apnea.

Physical control of breathing
Working together, the various control mechanisms regulate ventilation

to provide continuous airflow to the lungs. However, the amount of air that actually reaches the lungs with O_2 and then departs carrying CO_2 depends on lung volume and capacity, resistance to airflow, and compliance.

Effective gas exchange is opposed by three forces of resistance: elastic resistance, nonelastic (viscous) resistance, and airflow resistance. These forces can restrict respiration as well as add to the work of breathing.

Elastic resistance. The lung has a natural tendency to contract because of its tissue elasticity. This elasticity is derived partly from elastic fibers throughout the lung, which stretch during inspiration and spring back during expiration. But the elasticity is derived primarily from surface tension of the fluid lining the individual alveoli, which constantly promotes alveolar collapse. Two forces counter lung elasticity—chest wall rigidity combined with pleural fluid tension, and surfactant secretion in the alveoli, which reduces alveolar surface tension. (For more information, see *What happens during inspiration and expiration.*)

During inspiration, the cohesive force of the fluid between the visceral and parietal pleurae, combined with negative intrapleural pressure, causes the lung to expand with the chest wall. During expiration, these factors halt lung deflation at the chest wall's point of maximum contraction. The lung and chest wall function smoothly as a counterbalanced unit—as long as the pleurae remain intact. But when the pleurae are disturbed, such as by external puncture or rupture of a bleb, this pleural force of attraction is broken and lung collapse results, as in pneumothorax.

In the alveoli, surfactant coats the lining and prevents fluid contact with alveolar air. This creates a surface tension 2 to 14 times less than the fluid-air tension and reduces the tendency for alveolar collapse. Any disorder that interferes with surfactant production promotes lung collapse.

Nonelastic (viscous) resistance. This results from the force exerted on the thorax by the diaphragm and the abdominal contents, which inhibits the thorax from expanding downward. Not usually sufficient to compromise inspiration, this resistance becomes a problem in such conditions as obesity, abdominal distention, ascites, and late-term pregnancy.

Airflow resistance. This resistance derives from a change in airway radius or airflow pattern. Airway radius, a critical factor, decreases as large bronchi branch out through the lung. The radius also decreases when secretions accumulate in the bronchi or when condensation develops in ventilator tubing. A 50% reduction in airway radius causes a sixteenfold increase in resistance to airflow.

For the patient on a ventilator, airway length also becomes a factor. The ventilator tubing represents an extension of the tracheobronchial tree. And this extension directly affects airflow resistance—doubling the length, for instance, doubles the resistance. Understanding this principle will help you remember the strict limitations on ventilator tubing length.

The pattern of airflow—laminar, turbulent, or transitional—also affects resistance. (See *Understanding airflow patterns,* page 12.) Laminar flow offers minimal resis-

What happens during inspiration and expiration

These illustrations and descriptions explain how mechanical forces, such as the movement of intercostal muscles and the diaphragm, produce inspiration and expiration. A + indicates positive pressure; a − indicates negative pressure.

At rest

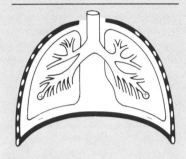

• The inspiratory muscles relax.
• Atmospheric pressure is maintained in the tracheobronchial tree while the lungs are at rest.
• No air movement occurs.

During inspiration

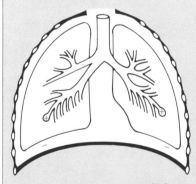

• The central nervous system (CNS) transmits impulses to the diaphragm via the phrenic nerve, stimulating contraction.
• The diaphragm descends as it contracts, enlarging the thorax vertically;

external intercostal muscles also contract (especially during deep or forced inspiration), raising the ribs and sternum and enlarging the thorax horizontally.
• Thoracic expansion lowers intrapleural pressure; pleural cohesion causes the lungs to expand with the thorax; lung expansion lowers the intrapulmonic (bronchoalveolar) pressure below atmospheric pressure.
• The intrapulmonic-atmospheric pressure gradient pulls air into the lungs until the two pressures equalize.

During expiration

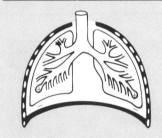

• CNS impulses to the diaphragm cease; the diaphragm slowly relaxes and moves up in the thorax, and the lungs recoil to their resting size and position.
• This recoil (usually passive, but aided during deep or forced expiration by CNS-stimulated contraction of internal intercostal muscles) also reduces the thorax to its resting size.
• Compression of the lungs and thorax causes intrapulmonic pressure to rise above atmospheric pressure.
• The intrapulmonic-atmospheric pressure gradient forces air out of the lungs until the two pressures equalize.

Understanding airflow patterns

Respiratory airflow occurs in three basic patterns: laminar, turbulent, and transitional.

Laminar flow
This linear pattern, which occurs primarily in the small peripheral airways, produces minimal airflow resistance.

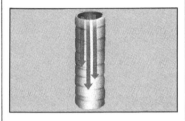

Turbulent flow
This eddying pattern results in increased airflow resistance. Typically, it occurs in the trachea and large central bronchi.

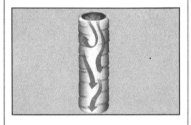

Transitional flow
This mixed airflow pattern occurs in the larger airways, especially where they branch or narrow because of an obstruction.

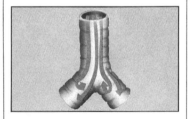

tance to airflow. The smooth angles in the small airways of the bronchial tree produce this desirable flow pattern.

Turbulent flow creates added friction, increasing resistance. Normal in the trachea and larger bronchi, turbulent flow may also occur in the smaller airways as a result of bronchoconstriction or excessive secretions. In a patient on a ventilator, condensation in the tubing also can change the flow pattern. Keep in mind that high airflow rates also induce turbulence and thus require higher pressures to deliver a normal tidal volume.

A mix of patterns, called transitional flow, occurs around obstructions and at transitional points in the larger airways, such as branches.

Compliance. The reciprocal of elasticity, compliance is the lung's ability to expand, yielding to intra-alveolar pressure during inspiration. Two factors influence compliance: chest wall expansibility and lung expansibility. Chest wall expansibility isn't routinely measured. That's because it's affected by skeletal muscle contraction, and valid measurement requires total muscle relaxation. In contrast, lung expansibility doesn't depend on physical relaxation for valid measurement.

The most common measurement, made under static conditions, static compliance is a product of the tidal volume divided by the pressure required to deliver that volume. This determines the change in volume occurring for every centimeter of water pressure (cm H_2O) increase. Normal static compliance is about 100 cc/cm H_2O.

Dynamic compliance is measured under nonstatic conditions, usually during inspiration. This measurement indicates the volume above which an increase in pressure won't significantly increase the volume of gas delivered. Normal dynamic compliance is 50 cc/cm H_2O.

Gas diffusion

All gas moves from an area of greater pressure to one of lesser pressure. During ventilation, the actions of the chest wall, pleurae, and lungs produce the changes in intrapulmonic and intrapleural pressure needed to move air into and out of the lungs. The next step in gas exchange – diffusion of O_2 into the blood and CO_2 out of it – occurs as the partial pressures of these gases on each side of the respiratory membrane create steep pressure gradients. (See *Understanding gas diffusion*, page 14.)

Rapid gas exchange. Normally, gas exchange takes place in half the time allowed for it. Blood is exposed to the respiratory membrane for about 0.8 second at rest. Virtually complete O_2 saturation of the blood occurs in half that time, and CO_2 exchange occurs 20 times faster than O_2 exchange. So, if a specific lung area receives an adequate volume of blood flow, the flow rate will not compromise gas exchange.

The speed of gas exchange and the specific pressure needed to effect the exchange depend on the solubility of gases in blood. Because CO_2 is much more soluble than O_2, it diffuses more rapidly and requires a much lower pressure gradient to do so, even when resistance to diffusion increases. If, for example, resistance increases because of a thickened respiratory membrane, CO_2 still may maintain its partial pressure and diffuse normally, whereas O_2 diffusion and partial pressure of oxygen (PO_2) decrease.

O_2 transport. Once diffusion occurs, arterial blood transports O_2 to the tissues in two ways: physically dissolved in plasma and chemically bound to hemoglobin. Plasma carries comparatively little O_2. Henry's law governs this relationship, stating that the amount of a gas dissolved in a liquid is directly proportional to the pressure of the gas against the liquid. So as gas pressure rises, the amount of gas that dissolves into the liquid to equalize that pressure differential also rises, depending on the solubility of the gas. Because O_2 resists dissolving in plasma, only about 3% is transported in this way.

Hemoglobin carries about 97% of the O_2 in the blood, depending on the PO_2 level. High PO_2, as occurs in pulmonary capillaries, causes O_2 to bind to the protein's ferrous iron (heme, or Fe^{++}) molecules to form oxyhemoglobin (HbO_2). Low PO_2, as found at the cellular level, reverses the bond, releasing O_2. (See *Oxyhemoglobin dissociation curve*, page 15.) Barriers to this bonding process include certain chemicals and carbon monoxide (CO). Chemicals such as nitrites convert hemoglobin to a ferric state (Fe^{+++}), called methemoglobin, making it incapable of combining with O_2. CO, which has an attraction to hemoglobin hundreds of times greater than that of O_2, easily displaces O_2 in the bonding process.

Hemoglobin bound to O_2 as completely as possible (normally about 1.34 cc O_2 per gram of hemoglobin) is considered 100% saturated. Less complete combinations are expressed as lower percentages. Saturation near 100% turns hemoglobin bright red, as with normal arterial blood. Desaturated hemoglobin, which is purple, produces the bluish tone of cyanosis. This sign,

Understanding gas diffusion

The concept of diffusion draws on Dalton's law of partial pressures. This law states that in a mixture of gases, the pressure (tension) exerted by each gas is independent of the other gases and directly corresponds to the percentage of the total mixture that it represents.

Here's how Dalton's law works: Atmospheric air inspired at sea level exerts a pressure of 760 mm Hg against all parts of the body. Oxygen represents 21% of air and thus exerts a partial pressure (PO_2) of 158 mm Hg, or 21% of 760 mm Hg. Carbon dioxide, a trace element of atmospheric air, has a partial pressure (PCO_2) of 0.3 mm Hg. Nitrogen, making up 78% of air, has a partial pressure (PN_2) of 596 mm Hg. Lastly, water vapor has a partial pressure (PH_2O) of 5.7 mm Hg.

During inspiration, the upper respiratory tract warms and humidifies atmospheric air, increasing the PH_2O to 47 mm Hg. Partial pressures of the other gases decline because total pressure must remain at 760 mm Hg.

Before entering the alveoli, inspired air mixes with gas that wasn't exhaled on the previous expiration. Because this gas contains more carbon dioxide and less oxygen than inspired air, partial pressures change again.

The air that finally enters the alveoli for diffusion across the respiratory membrane goes through further partial pressure changes. But this air remains high in oxygen pressure and low in carbon dioxide pressure. On the other side of the respiratory membrane is deoxygenated blood from the right ventricle, which has a low oxygen pressure and high carbon dioxide pressure.

The differential in partial pressures of oxygen and carbon dioxide causes the two gases to cross the respiratory membrane toward the lower side of their respective pressure gradients. Oxygen diffuses into the blood and carbon dioxide diffuses outward, equalizing the gas pressures on both sides of the respiratory membrane.

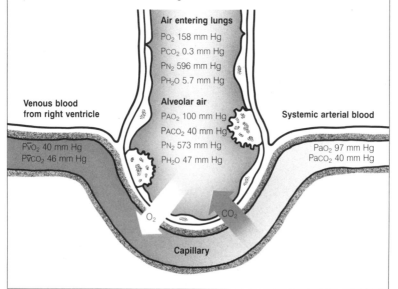

Air entering lungs
PO_2 158 mm Hg
PCO_2 0.3 mm Hg
PN_2 596 mm Hg
PH_2O 5.7 mm Hg

Venous blood from right ventricle

Alveolar air
PAO_2 100 mm Hg
$PACO_2$ 40 mm Hg
PN_2 573 mm Hg
PH_2O 47 mm Hg

Systemic arterial blood

$P\overline{v}O_2$ 40 mm Hg
$P\overline{v}CO_2$ 46 mm Hg

PaO_2 97 mm Hg
$PaCO_2$ 40 mm Hg

O_2

CO_2

Capillary

Oxyhemoglobin dissociation curve

The oxyhemoglobin dissociation curve depicts hemoglobin saturation (affinity for oxygen) at any PO_2. Note that the curve flattens out at a PO_2 of about 75 mm Hg; at this level, most of the hemoglobin is saturated, and an increase in PO_2 won't greatly improve saturation. Note, too, that when PO_2 falls below 60 mm Hg, rapid and extensive desaturation can occur, resulting in hypoxia.

Factors that alter hemoglobin's affinity and shift the curve include pH, PCO_2, and temperature. A rise in pH, or a drop in PCO_2 or temperature, induces hemoglobin to bond with oxygen, producing higher saturation at a given PO_2 and shifting the curve to the left. But these same factors inhibit oxygen release at the cellular level. Conversely, a drop in pH, or a rise in PCO_2 or temperature, induces hemoglobin to release oxygen, producing lower saturation at a given PO_2 and shifting the curve to the right. But these factors also inhibit hemoglobin bonding in the lungs.

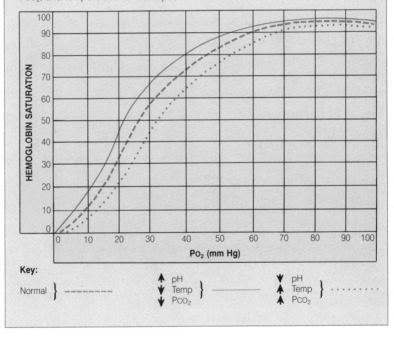

Key:

Normal } – – – – –

↑ pH
↓ Temp } ————
↓ PCO_2

↓ pH
↑ Temp } · · · · · · ·
↑ PCO_2

however, provides an unreliable indicator of hypoxemia because it doesn't appear until at least 5 g/dl of hemoglobin are desaturated — a condition that's more serious for an anemic patient with total hemoglobin of only 8 g/dl than for a polycythemic patient with total hemoglobin of 20 g/dl.

Once O_2-laden arterial blood reaches body tissues, internal respiration — gas exchange between systemic capillaries and interstitial fluid — occurs along pressure gradients. The O_2 moves into the interstitial fluid to nourish the cells, and

CO_2 leaves the fluid to travel in the blood. At this point, blood moves across the capillaries from the arterial to the venous system to begin its journey to the lungs, where the waste CO_2 is exchanged for O_2.

CO_2 transport. Blood carries CO_2 to the lungs in three ways: as a gas dissolved in plasma, coupled with hemoglobin as carbaminohemoglobin, and combined with water as carbonic acid (H_2CO_3) and its component ions. Only 7% is carried in blood plasma. Some of this 7% has a measurable partial pressure; the rest reacts very slowly with water to form carbonic acid, which, in reversible processes, may break down further into hydrogen ions (H^+) and bicarbonate ions (HCO_3^-).

About 23% of the CO_2 reacts faster with hemoglobin in the red blood cells (RBCs), forming the compound carbaminohemoglobin.

About 70% of the CO_2 converts to H_2CO_3 in the RBCs, a process occurring in a fraction of a second in the presence of the catalyzing enzyme carbonic anhydrase. With equal speed, the H_2CO_3 breaks down into hydrogen ions and bicarbonate ions. The hydrogen ions remain cell-bound, neutralized by the hemoglobin, and the bicarbonate ions trade places with chloride ions in the surrounding plasma. In this process, called chloride shift, the RBCs expel excess bicarbonate yet remain electrically neutral.

When venous blood enters the lung for gas exchange, all reversible chemical processes reverse, reforming CO_2. The gas diffuses into the alveoli for expiration.

Ventilation-perfusion ratio

How much O_2 and CO_2 trade places in the alveoli depends largely on the amount of O_2 the lungs can draw in and the amount of blood available in the lungs to oppose it. This ratio of ventilation to perfusion ($\dot{V}/\dot{Q}$ ratio) determines the effectiveness of gas exchange.

In the ideal model for gas exchange, the amount of air in the alveoli (ventilation) matches the amount of blood in the capillaries (perfusion), and gas exchange occurs easily along complementary pressure gradients. In reality, however, the match is unequal. The alveoli receive air at a rate of about 4 liters/minute, but the capillaries supply blood at a rate of about 5 liters/minute — creating a ventilation/perfusion ($\dot{V}/\dot{Q}$) mismatch of 4:5 or 0.8.

This ratio represents an average; it's not constant throughout the lung. Gravitational force makes ventilation relatively greater at the apex of the lung and blood flow greater at the base. Thus, alveoli at the apex are underperfused in relation to ventilation, resulting in a $\dot{V}/\dot{Q}$ ratio of about 3.0. This ratio gradually reverses down through the lung. The alveoli at the base are overperfused in relation to ventilation, for a $\dot{V}/\dot{Q}$ ratio of about 0.6.

Thus, an unequal pattern of gas exchange exists throughout the lung. Because of reduced blood flow, the Po_2 at the apex is more than 40 mm Hg lower than the Po_2 at the base. Exercise increases apical perfusion and, as a result, apical O_2 uptake.

Pathophysiology

Your ability to interpret clinical findings for specific disorders and to provide appropriate respiratory support depends on your knowledge of respiratory pathophysiology. This last section of the chapter explains the basic mechanisms of respiratory disorders that you need to understand.

Ineffective gas exchange

A central problem in respiratory disorders, ineffective gas exchange between the alveoli and the pulmonary capillaries can affect all body systems. For effective gas exchange, ventilation and perfusion must match as closely as possible. A $\dot{V}/\dot{Q}$ mismatch — resulting from ventilation-perfusion dysfunction or altered lung mechanics — accounts for most of the impaired gas exchange in respiratory disorders.

Ventilation-perfusion abnormalities. When ineffective gas exchange results from a physiologic abnormality, the result may be reduced ventilation to a lung unit (shunt), reduced perfusion to a unit (dead-space ventilation), or both (silent unit). (See *Understanding shunt and dead-space air,* at right, and *Basics of ventilation and perfusion,* page 18.)

The term shunting refers to the movement of unoxygenated blood to the left side of the heart. An abnormal shunt may occur from a physical defect that allows unoxygenated blood to bypass fully functioning alveoli. Or such a shunt may result when an airway obstruction prevents O_2 from reaching an adequately perfused area of the lung.

Keep in mind that a physical shunt occurs in the normal lung. The pulmonary veins collect O_2-depleted blood from the bronchial artery, which perfuses the bronchi, and from the thebesian veins, which drain the heart muscle. Shunting of this poorly oxygenated blood into arterial blood depresses arterial

Understanding shunt and dead-space air

The following definitions explain three key terms — shunt, dead-space air, and physiologic dead-space air.

Shunt: Area of the lung that is perfused but not ventilated. A shunt usually affects gas exchange in the alveoli. This abnormality commonly occurs in adult respiratory distress syndrome.

Dead-space air: Air contained in the conducting airways. This includes air in the nose, mouth, pharynx, larynx, trachea, and bronchial tree, but not the alveoli. The average amount of dead-space air is 150 ml for an adult male and 110 ml for an adult female.

Physiologic dead-space air: The sum of dead-space air and air in any nonfunctioning or partly functioning alveoli. Such defective alveoli, no longer active in gas exchange, may be adequately ventilated but may also lack good blood supply. This abnormality commonly occurs in pulmonary embolism.

PO_2, but not significantly for a person who has normal cardiac function. A person who has heart disease, however, also may have a physical defect between the right and left sides of the heart, which diverts greater amounts of unoxygenated blood directly into the arterial flow, seriously depressing arterial PO_2.

Respiratory disorders commonly are classified as shunt-producing if the $\dot{V}/\dot{Q}$ ratio falls below 0.8 or dead space–producing if the $\dot{V}/\dot{Q}$ ratio exceeds 0.8.

Changes in mechanics. Ineffective gas exchange also can result from

Basics of ventilation and perfusion

Effective gas exchange depends on the relationship between ventilation and perfusion ($\dot{V}/\dot{Q}$ ratio). The diagrams below show what happens when the $\dot{V}/\dot{Q}$ ratio is normal and abnormal.

Normal ventilation and perfusion
When ventilation and perfusion are matched, deoxygenated blood in the pulmonary artery enters the respiratory unit, then emerges oxygenated into the pulmonary vein.

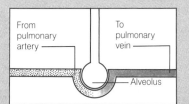

Inadequate ventilation (shunt)
When the $\dot{V}/\dot{Q}$ ratio is low, alveolar collapse causes hypoxemia. This usually results from acute diseases, such as atelectasis, pneumonia, and adult respiratory distress syndrome.

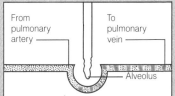

Inadequate perfusion (dead-space ventilation)
When the $\dot{V}/\dot{Q}$ ratio is high, as in the unit shown here, the alveolus receives inadequate blood flow. Note the narrowed capillary, indicating poor perfusion. This commonly results from a perfusion defect, such as pulmonary embolism or a disorder that decreases cardiac output.

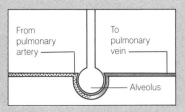

Inadequate ventilation and perfusion (silent unit)
The silent unit shown here has poor perfusion and ventilation. By diverting blood flow to better-ventilated lung areas, the silent unit helps compensate for a $\dot{V}/\dot{Q}$ imbalance. A silent unit can stem from several causes, including pulmonary embolism and chronic alveolar collapse.

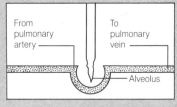

changes in lung mechanics that demand higher internal pressures to produce adequate breath volumes. This increases the work of breathing and reduces the effectiveness of gas exchange. These mechanical changes are categorized as either changes in compliance or changes in resistance.

• *Changes in compliance.* Changes in the ability to expand can occur in either the lung or the chest wall. Destruction of the lung's elastic fibers, as occurs in emphysema, increases lung compliance. The lung expands easily during inspiration but contracts with difficulty, increasing the work of breathing during expiration. Lung compliance usually remains normal in chronic bronchitis and bronchial asthma because airway spasm (rather than a change in the lung's cellular structure) creates the obstruction to airflow. However, compliance decreases in interstitial and alveolar pulmonary diseases — such as pulmonary edema, pulmonary fibrosis, and sarcoidosis — because characteristic cellular changes make inspiration more difficult.

Chest wall compliance may be affected by thoracic deformity, muscle spasm, or abdominal distention. Compliance may decrease in ankylosing spondylitis, kyphosis, marked obesity, extreme pectus excavatum, scoliosis, and disorders causing muscle spasticity.

• *Changes in resistance.* Changes in the pressure needed to produce airflow may occur in the lung tissue, as with sarcoidosis and other interstitial lung diseases; in the chest wall, as with pleurisy and other pleural disorders; or in the airways. This third type accounts for about 80% of all respiratory system resistance. Airway resistance typically increases in obstructive diseases, such as asthma, chronic bronchitis, and emphysema. Thus, the work of breathing, particularly during expiration, increases to compensate for narrowed airways and diminished gas exchange.

Signs of ineffective gas exchange.
Ineffective gas exchange eventually results in hypoxia (tissue O_2 deficiency). Hypoxia, which may occur at any point from ventilation to transport to cell metabolism, results in O_2 deficiency at the cellular level. Such a decrease in cellular O_2 concentration means the cell must resort to anaerobic metabolism to supply its energy needs. That leads to lactic acidosis.

The mechanisms of hypoxia vary because O_2 delivery to the cells depends on the blood's O_2-carrying capacity, cardiac output, and peripheral blood flow. For example, insufficient hemoglobin (as in anemia) reduces the blood's ability to transport adequate O_2. A decreased blood volume (as in severe hemorrhage) also reduces the amount of blood that's available to transport O_2 to the cells. The following list classifies hypoxia according to physiologic pathways:

• hypoxic (anoxic or arterial) hypoxia — deficient oxygenation of arterial blood despite its normal O_2-carrying capacity, possibly resulting from airway obstruction

• anemic hypoxia — reduced blood O_2-carrying capacity resulting from hemoglobin deficiency

• stagnant (circulatory) hypoxia — normal blood O_2-carrying capacity but inadequate tissue oxygenation because of vascular obstruction and reduced capillary blood flow

• histotoxic (metabolic) hypoxia — normal blood PO_2, but inadequate tissue oxygenation because of impaired oxidative-enzyme cellular mechanisms that prevent cells from metabolizing O_2. Such hypoxia is particularly acute if the cell's demand for O_2 is excessively high.

Other signs of ineffective gas exchange include:

• hypoxemia — a decrease in the O_2 concentration of arterial blood (this term is commonly used incorrectly as a synonym for hypoxia)

• hypocapnia — decreased CO_2 concentration in the blood

• hypercapnia — increased blood retention of CO_2.

Compensatory mechanisms

Ineffective gas exchange has an additional implication beyond poor tissue oxygenation: It also promotes CO_2 retention and threatens homeostasis by upsetting the systemic acid-base balance. Fortunately, physiologic compensatory mechanisms usually can blunt this toxic effect before it stresses other body systems.

Normally, the body's acid-base balance remains within a very narrow pH range of 7.35 to 7.45. An acute drop to 7.25 (acidosis) or rise to 7.55 (alkalosis) may be life-threatening. The pH will drop when too many hydrogen ions are produced; conversely, the pH will rise when too many bicarbonate ions are produced.

Body fluids fluctuate constantly, their composition altered by acids, CO_2, and water from cellular metabolism of carbohydrates, proteins, and fats. CO_2 and water unite to form carbonic acid, which dissociates into hydrogen ions and bicarbonate ions. Three regulatory mechanisms neutralize or eliminate excessive hydrogen or bicarbonate ions and maintain the body's normal pH: acid-base buffers, the respiratory system itself, and the renal system.

Acid-base buffers. These pairs of weak acids and related bases operate within seconds to reduce the danger of stronger incoming acids and bases. By combining with a strong acid, which would dissociate to yield many hydrogen ions and thus sharply lower the pH, these buffers create a weaker acid that dissociates into fewer hydrogen ions and has a gentler effect on pH. They react similarly to neutralize a strong base, thereby keeping pH fluctuations to a minimum.

The major buffers of body fluids include bicarbonates, phosphates, and proteins, such as hemoglobin. The bicarbonates are mainly responsible for buffering blood and interstitial fluid. Among the buffers, the bicarbonates alone have a limitless outlet in the respiratory system to reduce acidity and renew themselves through increased CO_2 expiration.

Respiratory regulation. The second compensatory mechanism, the respiratory system normally can restore homeostasis within minutes. Because the amount of CO_2 in plasma determines the amount of carbonic acid and hydrogen ions produced, any rise in PCO_2 increases acidity, and any drop in PCO_2 increases alkalinity. Working together to sense and correct pH changes, the medullary respiratory centers and the lungs strive to maintain PCO_2 at 40 mm Hg — a level that facilitates pulmonary CO_2 excretion at a rate equalling cellular CO_2 production.

The medullary respiratory centers and lungs alter respiratory rate and depth to eliminate more or less CO_2 — and acid — as necessary to control pH. But when a respiratory disorder causes prolonged hyperventilation or hypoventilation, compensatory mechanisms may fail and respiratory alkalosis or acidosis results.

Renal regulation. The body's third and long-term regulator, the renal system intervenes when the first two compensatory mechanisms fail to correct pH imbalance. Within several hours or over several days, the kidneys adjust pH by excreting nonvolatile (fixed) acids — the acids the lungs can't excrete — and by either excreting hydrogen ions and reabsorbing bicarbonate ions to correct excess acidity or reversing this action to correct alkalosis.

In cases of metabolic acidosis or metabolic alkalosis, which stem from altered metabolic rather than respiratory patterns, renal and respiratory compensatory mechanisms work together. The kidneys adjust the levels of appropriate ions, while the lungs alter respiratory rate and depth to eliminate or conserve CO_2.

Thus, mechanisms exist to offset the effects of inefficient gas exchange. Compensation for acid-base imbalance involves a systemic shift in the opposite direction that moves pH back within normal limits. A primary respiratory imbalance produces an opposing compensatory metabolic response. For example, respiratory acidosis triggers conservation of bicarbonate ions and excretion of hydrogen ions (compensatory metabolic alkalosis).

But when disease or dysfunction interferes with compensatory mechanisms, a multisystemic problem requiring intervention may develop. For instance, a patient with chronic obstructive pulmonary disease who develops diabetic ketoacidosis can't compensate by increasing CO_2 expiration. Remember, too, that a patient with chronic respiratory disease will exhibit an elevated bicarbonate level as his kidneys compensate for CO_2 retention to maintain a normal pH. Correcting the elevated bicarbonate level only aggravates acidosis. Thus, when treating systemic dysfunction, you must address the primary problem, not the compensatory response.

Suggested readings

Guyton, A.C., ed. *Textbook of Medical Physiology,* 7th ed. Philadelphia: W.B. Saunders Co., 1986.

Kinney, M.R., et al. *AACN'S Clinical Reference for Critical Care Nursing,* 2nd ed. New York: McGraw-Hill Book Co., 1988.

Thibodeau, G., and Anthony, C.P. *Structure and Function of the Body.* St. Louis: C.V. Mosby Co., 1987.

Williams, P.L., et al, eds. *Gray's Anatomy,* 37th rev. ed. New York: Churchill, 1989.

2

RESPIRATORY ASSESSMENT

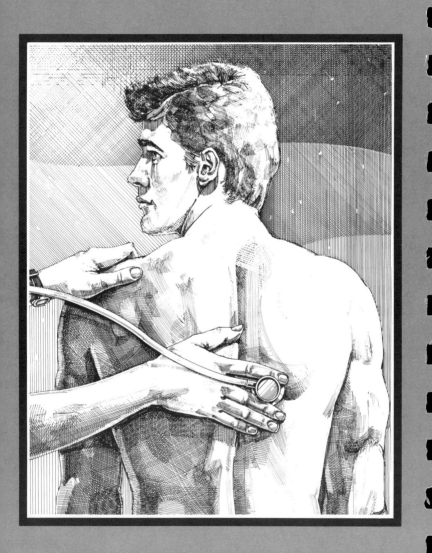

Patients receiving respiratory support require continuous monitoring and frequent assessment. Just how frequently — and how extensively — you assess such a patient will depend on his particular needs. With most patients, you'll probably perform a complete assessment only once a shift. But if your patient is receiving mechanical ventilation, you'll perform a brief assessment at least every 2 hours. And if the settings on his ventilator are changed, you may have to assess him every 5 to 15 minutes until you can determine his response.

Because almost all body systems can be affected by poor respiratory function, you need to assess more than just the respiratory system. For example, you should be alert for a change in your patient's level of consciousness (LOC) — an early sign of decreased oxygenation. Also, keep in mind that treatments aimed at correcting a patient's respiratory problem may affect other body functions. Mechanical ventilation, for instance, increases intrapulmonic and intrathoracic pressures, affecting ventricular filling and lowering cardiac output. Reduced cardiac output, in turn, decreases perfusion of the major organs, impairing their function. So you may have to routinely assess a particular organ or system.

To help you fine-tune your patient's respiratory therapy, you'll also monitor his arterial blood gases. To obtain an on-the-spot evaluation of his oxygenation status, you may use continuous mixed venous oxygen saturation ($S\bar{v}O_2$) monitoring, pulse oximetry, or capnography. What's more, you'll probably perform pulmonary function tests to evaluate his ventilatory status, and you may help with chest X-rays to evaluate anatomic abnormalities.

In this chapter, you'll learn how and when to perform all these procedures. First, though, review how to take a history and perform a thorough physical examination.

Health history

Typically, a complete health history will be obtained when a patient first seeks medical attention. This establishes a baseline and helps determine the cause of his illness, any factors that may influence treatment decisions, and the treatment plan. When you take a history during a patient's hospitalization, focus on his current symptoms or changes from the baseline.

Sometimes, you won't be able to obtain information from the patient. He may be unconscious or unable to communicate because of an artificial airway. In such cases, monitoring and evaluating your patient's condition and conferring with his family becomes critical.

Current history

If your patient can communicate, ask him about any signs or symptoms he's experiencing and how he feels now compared with when he first complained of his respiratory problem. Focus on the signs and symptoms that most often indicate respiratory dysfunction: cough, sputum production, dyspnea, and chest pain. Monitoring changes in these signs and symptoms will help you evaluate changes in your patient's condition, his response to treatment, and any complications. You'll also be able to determine how your patient is coping with his illness and if he thinks he's improving.

Cough. Ask your patient if he's coughing more or less than he did before. Does the cough change with any specific incident or activity— for instance, does it get worse after a respiratory treatment, when he sits up or lies down, during the day or at night, or when he takes a deep breath? Remember, the absence of a cough doesn't necessarily mean that the patient is improving. Sometimes a patient can't produce an effective cough because his ventilation is inadequate or a disorder has left him too weak, even though he has secretions or his airways are irritated. Also, an artificial airway may either override or stimulate the cough reflex. So the presence or absence of a cough in a patient with such a device can be misleading.

Sputum production. Does the patient's coughing produce sputum? If so, examine it. Does it appear frothy? What color is it? Has the color, consistency, or amount of sputum changed? If so, the primary disorder may be improving or worsening, or a secondary disorder or complication may have developed. A color change from white to yellow or green indicates infection. Blood-tinged or rust-colored sputum may be due to trauma from coughing, suctioning, or an underlying condition like bronchitis, pulmonary infarction or infection, tuberculosis, or a tumor. Does the sputum have an odor? Foul-smelling sputum may result from an anaerobic infection such as an abscess.

Dyspnea. Ask the patient if his shortness of breath is getting better or worse. Remember, dyspnea is subjective. A patient who has improved clinically may perceive that his dyspnea has worsened. A feeling of not being in control or anxiety about the illness can contribute to such a perception.

Find out if the dyspnea is continuous or if it changes with activity and circumstances. For example, does it get worse when the patient moves about or when visitors come or go? Does it require more or less activity for your patient to experience the same amount of breathlessness he has had before? Does anything relieve the dyspnea— perhaps a change in position, relaxation, medication, or use of oxygen?

If dyspnea is a new symptom, it could indicate either a worsening of the underlying condition or a new disorder. Nosocomial lung infections are common. So if dyspnea occurs or worsens in a patient with an underlying condition such as emphysema, he may have developed secondary pneumonia.

Chest pain. Is the chest pain a new symptom? If so, when did it begin? Is it associated with a specific activity or incident, such as movement, respiratory treatment, or anxiety? Have your patient describe the pain in his own words, but try to get specifics about its intensity, location, and duration. Ask if the pain radiates to any other part of his body. Is it accompanied by other signs and symptoms, such as coughing, sneezing, or shortness of breath? Does the pain occur during normal breathing or only with a deep breath? If it occurs only with a deep breath, the pain is pleuritic.

Chest pain isn't usually associated with lung disorders because the lungs have no pain-sensitive nerves. However, the parietal pleura and the tracheobronchial tree can sense pain, and conditions affecting these structures can be painful. A patient may also have chest pain of cardiac origin when poor oxygenation results in myocardial ischemia.

Physical examination

To perform a thorough and accurate physical examination, place the patient in a position that allows you access to his posterior and anterior chest. Also, make sure the lighting will allow you to detect changes in his skin color. As mentioned earlier, you'll usually have to make the full assessment described in this section only once a shift. However, depending on your patient's condition and its treatment, you may have to perform some parts of the assessment—monitoring vital signs, for instance—as often as every 5 minutes.

Positioning the patient
If your patient's condition permits, have him sit on the edge of a bed or examining table or in a chair, leaning slightly forward with his arms folded across his chest. If this isn't possible, place him in semi-Fowler's position for the anterior chest examination. Then ask him to lean forward slightly, using the side rails or mattress for support, so you can examine his posterior chest. If your patient can't lean forward for posterior chest examination, place him in a lateral position or request assistance from another staff member to help the patient sit up.

When you use the lateral position to examine your patient's posterior chest, both the mattress and organ displacement distort sounds and lung expansion. To compensate for these effects, examine the patient first on one side; then roll him on his other side and repeat the examination.

Your examination must cover three thoracic areas—posterior, anterior, and lateral. You can begin with any of these areas. And you may assess the lateral chest while the patient is positioned for either posterior or anterior examination. The sequence you choose isn't important; using it consistently is. So always proceed systematically, comparing one side of the chest with the other.

Monitoring vital signs
When evaluating a patient's vital signs, focus on the changes from his baseline rather than deviations from normal. For example, if your patient's respiratory rate was 40 breaths/minute on admission and it's now 28, you'd note his improvement, even though his respiratory rate is still above normal (12 to 20 breaths/minute).

Respirations. Monitor the patient continuously for signs and symptoms of severe hypoxia or acute respiratory difficulty. The body initially compensates for hypoxia by increasing the respiratory rate and depth. But when the body tires, respiratory rate and depth decrease. If any of the following develop suddenly (or if they worsen), your patient probably requires immediate intervention:
• change in LOC
• severe shortness of breath
• rapid, very deep or very shallow respirations, or slow respirations
• use of accessory muscles when breathing
• intercostal and sternal retractions
• cyanosis
• audible sounds (such as wheezing or stridor)
• diaphoresis

• nasal flaring
• extreme apprehension or agitation.

To determine the rate, rhythm, and depth of your patient's respirations, observe him at rest. Make sure he's unaware that you're counting his respirations. If he's conscious of his respirations, he may alter his natural pattern.

Count the patient's respirations for 1 minute to ensure accuracy. Counting for 15 seconds and multiplying by 4 increases the risk of an inaccurate reading, especially if the patient has an irregular breathing pattern. In patients with a respiratory disorder, this inaccuracy can be significant.

Observe the patient for rapid, shallow respirations (tachypnea); rapid, deep respirations (hyperpnea); very slow respirations (bradypnea); or an abnormal pattern of respirations, such as Cheyne-Stokes respirations (see *Recognizing common respiratory patterns*). Note whether the patient is breathing abdominally or thoracically. Men and children usually breathe abdominally; women, thoracically. Patients with chronic obstructive pulmonary disease (COPD) appear to breathe with their shoulders because their trapezius and sternocleidomastoid muscles are so hypertrophied. These patients also take longer than normal to exhale, sometimes reaching an inspiratory-expiratory ratio of 1:4. (The normal ratio is 1:2.)

If your patient is on a mechanical ventilator, his respiratory rate will be controlled by the machine. In certain modes, such as intermittent mandatory ventilation, the patient can initiate respirations above this rate. So when you're assessing respirations, check if your patient's breathing pattern is consistent with the mode selected. Make sure the machine is delivering the correct number of breaths per minute, that the patient is breathing with the machine and not against it (asynchronous breathing), and that the machine cycles appropriately when the patient initiates the breath.

Temperature. Illness puts added stress on the body that can result in fever. But usually, fever indicates an infection. And because patients with respiratory disorders tend to develop secondary lung infections, you need to monitor temperature.

A patient with an artificial airway runs a high risk of infection because the protective mechanisms that help prevent organisms from entering the lungs are bypassed. Central lines for monitoring, a tracheostomy tube, and an indwelling urinary catheter also increase the risk of secondary infection.

Dehydration can cause fever, too. So be sure to evaluate the patient's clinical signs to confirm that he's receiving appropriate treatment; if he has a fever from dehydration, he needs fluids, not antibiotics. No matter what the cause, fever increases the body's metabolic demands and oxygen needs, which can, in turn, affect a patient's respiratory needs.

Fever also affects the binding of oxygen to hemoglobin. An increase in temperature shifts the oxyhemoglobin dissociation curve to the right, decreasing oxygen saturation and increasing oxygen delivery to the tissues for a given partial pressure of oxygen in arterial blood (PaO_2). So you need to report a patient's temperature whenever you send for an ABG analysis.

Pulse. Monitor pulses to detect whether poor ventilation is affecting the patient's heart rate or if his

Recognizing common respiratory patterns

Use this chart as a guide for noting differences in respiratory rates, rhythms, and depths.

PATTERN	CHARACTERISTICS
Eupnea	Normal respiratory rate and rhythm. For adults and teenagers, 12 to 20 breaths/minute; for children ages 2 to 12, 20 to 30 breaths/minute; for neonates, 30 to 50 breaths/minute. Occasionally, deep breaths at a rate of 2 or 3 per minute.
Tachypnea	Increased respiratory rate, as seen in fever. Respiratory rate increases about 4 breaths/minute for every degree Fahrenheit above normal.
Bradypnea	Slower but regular respirations. Can occur when the brain's respiratory control center is affected by an opiate, a tumor, alcohol, a metabolic disorder, or respiratory decompensation. This pattern is normal during sleep.
Apnea	Absence of breathing. May be periodic.
Hyperpnea	Deeper, faster respirations.
Cheyne-Stokes respirations	Respirations gradually become faster and deeper than normal, then slower, over a 30- to 170-second period. Periods of apnea for 20 to 60 seconds.
Biot's respirations	Faster and deeper respirations than normal, with abrupt pauses. Each breath has same depth. May occur with spinal meningitis or other CNS conditions.
Kussmaul's respirations	Faster and deeper respirations without pauses; in adults, over 20 breaths/minute. Breathing usually sounds labored, with deep breaths that resemble sighs. Can occur with or result from renal failure or metabolic acidosis.
Apneustic breathing	Prolonged gasping inspiration, followed by extremely short, inefficient expiration. Can occur with or result from lesions in the brain's respiratory center.

heart rate is affecting perfusion. Hypoxia increases the pulse rate in response to sympathetic stimulation. Hypoxia can also cause cardiac arrhythmias if the myocardial oxygen supply is compromised — especially in a patient with underlying cardiac disease. An irregular pulse indicates an arrhythmia. A weak, thready, or irregular pulse can reflect decreased perfusion to the lungs and a worsening of the ventilation-perfusion ratio.

Blood pressure. This measurement can help determine if the patient is compensating for inadequate ventilation. With acute respiratory distress, blood pressure initially remains normal or rises slightly as a compensatory mechanism. During decompensation, it falls.

Assessing LOC

Because the brain needs large amounts of oxygenated blood to function properly, LOC provides a sensitive indicator of adequate oxygenation. Closely monitor your patient for such changes as lethargy, agitation, increased anxiety, somnolence, confusion, and irritability. Progressive deterioration indicates severe hypoxia. Remember, however, that hypoxia isn't the only cause of changes in LOC. Your patient may be irritable because of lack of sleep, for example. The extra work of breathing or the noise on the unit may have prevented him from getting restful sleep.

Inspecting the skin

Inspect your patient's skin color under natural light, if possible, because fluorescent light doesn't show true skin color. Look for cyanosis, remembering that:
• it's a late sign of hypoxia
• it may also result from vasocon-

striction and diminished blood flow
• severely anemic patients with respiratory difficulty don't appear cyanotic
• polycythemic patients may appear cyanotic and not be hypoxic because of their extra hemoglobin, which can't be saturated.

To determine the most likely cause of cyanosis, consider its location. *Central cyanosis* reflects excessive amounts of unsaturated hemoglobin in arterial blood. This can result from inadequate oxygenation, right-to-left cardiac shunting, or a hematologic disorder. Look for central cyanosis in highly vascular areas: the lips, nail beds, tip of the nose, ear helices, and underside of the tongue. With dark-skinned patients, inspect those areas where cyanotic changes would be apparent, such as the mucous membranes.

Peripheral cyanosis, only apparent in the nail beds and sometimes on the lips, reflects sluggish peripheral circulation caused by vasoconstriction, reduced cardiac output, or vascular obstruction. Under these conditions, peripheral tissues remove increased amounts of oxygen from the blood, causing reduced venous oxygen saturation.

Look for flushing, which can indicate increased partial pressure of carbon dioxide in arterial blood ($PaCO_2$). Diaphoresis may signal fever or infection, or may result from anxiety or a pulmonary disorder.

To evaluate the skin for turgor, pinch a fold of skin. When you let go, the skin should return to its original position immediately. If it doesn't, the finding is known as tenting — an indication of interstitial dehydration. Tenting may be normal in an elderly patient.

Assessing the face and neck

Observe your patient's face for signs

of respiratory distress, such as nasal flaring. If he has a nasally inserted endotracheal tube or a nasal oxygen cannula, inspect the skin around the nostrils for redness or excoriation. If the patient has a tracheostomy tube, examine the skin around the tracheostomy for signs of infection. Make sure that the tracheostomy or endotracheal tube is secure to prevent accidental extubation.

Palpate the patient's neck for crepitus, which could indicate air leaking into the subcutaneous tissues. Examine his oropharynx for color changes such as cyanosis; white patches, possibly indicating *Candida* infection; inflammation; and ulcerations, bleeding, exudate, or lesions — particularly around the oral airways or orally inserted endotracheal tube. Remember that a dark-skinned patient will normally have dark patches on the mucous membranes.

Observe whether the patient's trachea is in the midline position. Also, check again for accessory neck muscle use. If you can't see the trachea, palpate to determine its position (see *Palpating tracheal position*). If the patient has tracheal deviation and shows other signs of respiratory distress, he may have a tension pneumothorax — a life-threatening emergency requiring immediate intervention.

Also observe and palpate his neck over the trachea for swelling, bruises, tenderness, and masses that might obstruct breathing.

Inspecting the chest

To establish a baseline, begin your examination of the chest by inspecting for drainage, open wounds, bruises, abrasions, scars, cuts, and punctures, as well as for rib deformities, fractures, lesions, or masses.

Palpating tracheal position

To find the trachea, place the fingertips of one hand at the middle base of the patient's lower jaw. Then gently slide your fingertips down the center of his neck to locate the larynx. You should be able to feel the trachea in the area of the sternal notch.

Now assess for tracheal position. Place an index finger or thumb along each side of the trachea. Then note the distance between each side and the corresponding sternocleidomastoid muscle. The distance on the two sides should be equal.

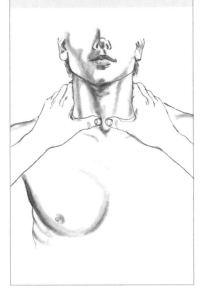

If the patient has a chest tube or central catheter in place or has a suture line from thoracic surgery, also examine the incision sites for signs of infection.

Observe the shape of the chest wall. Compare the anteroposterior diameter of the chest to the transverse diameter. The normal ratio of these diameters is between 1:2 and 5:7. This ratio increases in patients who have COPD or osteoporosis with kyphosis. Also note any chest deformities that can interfere with chest expansion, such as pectus excavatum, pectus carinatum, or scoliosis.

Next, watch your patient's chest movement during respirations. Normally, the chest moves upward and outward symmetrically on inspiration. Impaired movement may occur when pain, poor positioning, or abdominal distention causes restricted chest wall expansion. Paradoxical movement of the chest wall may result from fractured ribs or flail chest.

If your patient is on a ventilator, observe how his chest movements coincide with the inspiratory phase of the ventilator. Asynchronous movements may result from insufficient ventilation or from anxiety possibly caused by pain, fear, air hunger, or increased intracranial pressure.

Check for accessory muscle use and retraction of intercostal spaces during inspiration, which can indicate respiratory distress. Sudden, violent intercostal retraction indicates airway obstruction or tension pneumothorax. In some obstructive disorders like COPD, abdominal muscles retract during expiration as the patient attempts to force air from the alveoli. Inspiratory intercostal bulging can occur with cardiac enlargement and aneurysm; localized expiratory bulging occurs with rib fractures and flail chest.

Palpating the chest

Using your finger joints and fingerpads, gently palpate the entire chest to identify the thoracic structures that'll help you determine the approximate locations of the lung lobes (see *Locating thoracic landmarks*). If your patient is a woman, you may have to move her breasts so you can palpate the anterior chest.

Usually, the apices are located about ¾" to 1½" (2 to 4 cm) above the inner aspect of the clavicles. The inferior border of the lower lobes is located at the 10th thoracic spinous process; on full inspiration, it may descend to the 12th thoracic spinous process. To locate the lower lung borders in a patient lying laterally, palpate the visible free-floating ribs or costal margins; then count four intercostal spaces upward for the general location of the lower lung fields (see *Locating lung lobes*, pages 32 and 33).

While palpating, note any retractions or bulging in the intercostal spaces, indicating increased inspiratory or expiratory effort; any areas of tenderness over the ribs, possibly indicating a fracture, costochondritis, or a tumor; and crepitus (especially around wound sites, central lines, a tracheostomy tube, or a chest tube), indicating air leaking into subcutaneous tissues.

Palpate the slope of the ribs. Normally, they slope downward. But in a patient with an increased anteroposterior diameter from an obstructive lung disease, you'll palpate ribs that are abnormally horizontal.

Thoracic expansion. To palpate for symmetrical thoracic expansion (respiratory expansion), place your palms — fingers together and thumbs abducted toward the spine — flat on the bilateral sections of your patient's lower posterior chest wall. Position your thumbs at the 10th rib level, and lightly grasp his lateral rib cage with your hands. As the patient inhales, his posterior chest should move upward and outward, and your thumbs should move apart

Locating thoracic landmarks

These illustrations highlight the key thoracic landmarks of the posterior, anterior, and lateral chest.

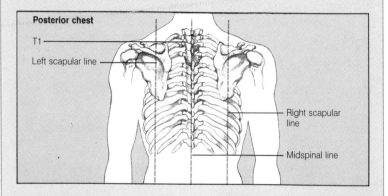

Posterior chest

- T1
- Left scapular line
- Right scapular line
- Midspinal line

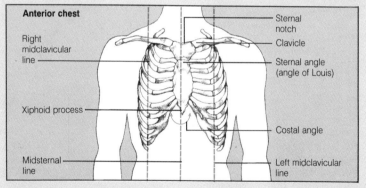

Anterior chest

- Right midclavicular line
- Xiphoid process
- Midsternal line
- Sternal notch
- Clavicle
- Sternal angle (angle of Louis)
- Costal angle
- Left midclavicular line

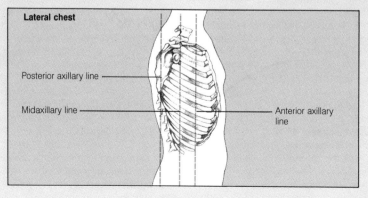

Lateral chest

- Posterior axillary line
- Midaxillary line
- Anterior axillary line

Locating lung lobes

Use the thoracic landmarks to help you locate a patient's lung lobes from the posterior, left lateral, right lateral, and anterior views.

Posterior view. The oblique fissures divide the upper lobes from the lower lobes of both lungs. You can approximate the location of these fissures by imagining bilateral lines drawn laterally and inferiorly from the third thoracic spinous process to the inferior border of the scapula. Note that you can identify only two lobes in each lung in the posterior view.

Left lateral view. The left oblique fissure divides the left upper lobe (LUL) from the left lower lobe (LLL). You can estimate the location of this fissure by imagining a line drawn anteriorly and inferiorly from the third thoracic spinous process to the sixth rib at the midclavicular line.

Right lateral view. You can determine the location of the right oblique fissure as you did for the left oblique fissure. But the right oblique fissure divides

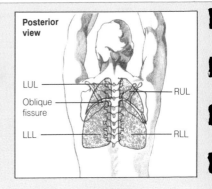

Posterior view

LUL
Oblique fissure
LLL
RUL
RLL

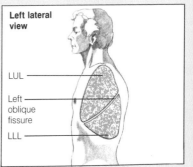

Left lateral view

LUL
Left oblique fissure
LLL

equally. When he exhales, your thumbs should return to midline and touch each other again.

Next, on the anterior chest, place your thumbs along the costal margins, pointing toward the xiphoid process, with your hands along the lateral rib cage. Ask your patient to inhale deeply, and observe for symmetrical thoracic expansion.

Unequal thoracic expansion could indicate pleural effusion, atelectasis, pulmonary embolus, or fractured ribs or sternum. Also, if an endotracheal tube has been inserted too far and has entered the right mainstem bronchus, the sides of the chest will expand unequally.

Mechanical ventilation can affect thoracic expansion, so take the type of ventilation into account when assessing these patients. Positive end-expiratory pressure (PEEP), for instance, may make thoracic expansion less pronounced because it keeps alveoli partially expanded during expiration. Independent or differential lung ventilation delivers a different tidal volume and level of PEEP to each lung, changing the shape of chest movement. And you won't see any significant thoracic expansion in a patient receiving high-frequency ventilation, making this assessment useless in such patients.

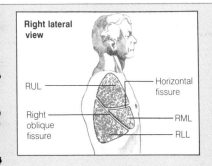

Right lateral view

RUL

Right oblique fissure

Horizontal fissure

RML

RLL

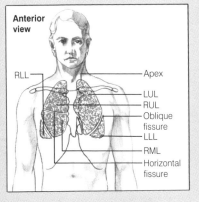

Anterior view

RLL

Apex

LUL

RUL

Oblique fissure

LLL

RML

Horizontal fissure

the upper portion of the lung (both upper and middle lobes) from the right lower lobe (RLL). To approximate the division of the right upper lobe (RUL) and the right middle lobe (RML), imagine a line drawn medially from the fifth rib at the midaxillary line to the fourth rib at the midclavicular line.

Anterior view. The apices lie ¾″ to 1½″ (2 to 4 cm) above the inner portion of the clavicle. The inferior borders run from the sixth rib at the midclavicular line to the eighth rib at the midaxillary line.

The horizontal fissure divides the RUL from the RML. You can approximate this fissure by imagining a line drawn anteriorly and superiorly from the fifth rib at the midaxillary line to the fourth rib at the midclavicular line.

The right oblique fissure divides the RLL from the RML; the left oblique fissure divides the LLL from the LUL. You can estimate the location of these fissures by imagining lines drawn medially and inferiorly from the fifth rib at the midaxillary line to the sixth rib at the midclavicular line.

Tactile fremitus. To palpate for tactile fremitus, follow the recommended palpation sequence (see *Sequences for palpation,* page 34). Place the top portion of your palms on the chest wall, and ask your patient to say "99." Palpable vibrations will be transmitted from his bronchopulmonary system along the solid surfaces of his chest wall to your palms.

Note the symmetry of the vibrations and the areas of increased, decreased, or absent fremitus. Fremitus will be most pronounced in areas of increased airflow—for example, where the trachea . branches into the right and left

mainstem bronchi in the upper lobes—and less noticeable in the lower regions of the thorax. You'll also find increased fremitus in areas of lung consolidation, such as occur with pneumonia or atelectasis.

Fremitus will be decreased or absent over the precordium, areas of decreased airflow, and areas of increased distance between the lung and your hand. Expect to find decreased fremitus also over the lung bases, in obese patients, and in those with such conditions as emphysema, pleural effusion, hemothorax, pneumothorax, and pulmonary fibrosis.

Palpating for fremitus also allows

Sequences for palpation

Follow the sequences illustrated here to palpate the posterior and anterior chest.

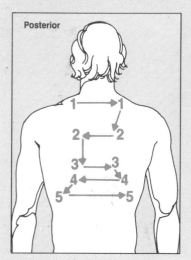

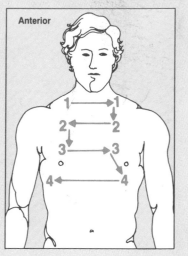

you to estimate the level of the diaphragm. Place the ulnar side of your extended hand on the posterior chest wall parallel to the expected diaphragm level. Then ask your patient to say "99" as you move your hand downward. The level at which you no longer feel fremitus indicates the approximate diaphragm level.

Percussing the chest

To determine more precisely the location, as well as the density, of the lungs and diaphragm, you'll need to percuss the patient's chest, following the standard sequence (see *Percussion and auscultation sequences*). Assess for five types of percussion sounds: flat, dull, resonant, hyperresonant, and tympanic (see *Understanding percussion sounds,* page 36).

Start by percussing the patient's posterior chest across the top of each shoulder. The area overlying the lung apices — approximately 2″ (5 cm) — should be resonant. Then percuss downward toward the diaphragm at 2″ intervals, comparing the right and left sides as you proceed. The posterior chest should produce resonance, except over the bony areas. At the level of the diaphragm, resonance should change to dullness.

On the anterior chest, begin percussing at the supraclavicular areas, again moving downward and comparing the right and left sides. You should hear resonance until you reach the third or fourth intercostal space (ICS) to the left of the sternum, where you'll hear a dull sound produced by the heart. This sound should continue as you percuss down toward the fifth ICS and laterally toward the midclavicular line

Percussion and auscultation sequences

Follow the percussion and auscultation sequences shown here to help you identify abnormalities in your patient's lungs. Remember to compare sounds from one side to the other as you proceed. Document any abnormal sounds you hear and describe them carefully, including their location.

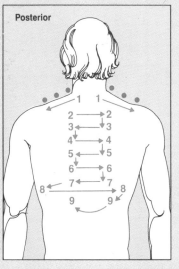

Posterior

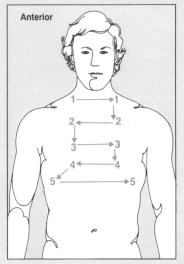

Anterior

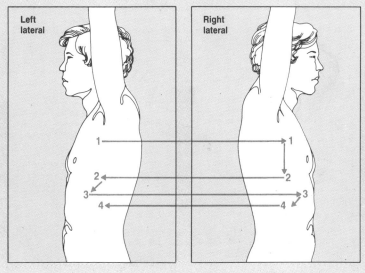

Left lateral

Right lateral

Understanding percussion sounds

SOUND	PITCH	INTENSITY	QUALITY	IMPLICATIONS
Flatness	High	Soft	Extreme dullness	Normal over sternum. Over lung may indicate atelectasis, pleural effusion.
Dullness	Medium	Medium	Thudlike	Normal over liver, heart, diaphragm. Over lung may indicate pneumonia, tumor, atelectasis, pleural effusion.
Resonance	Low	Moderate to loud	Hollow	Normal over lung.
Hyperresonance	Lower than resonance	Very loud	Booming	Normal over child's lung. Over adult lung may indicate emphysema, chronic bronchitis, asthma, pneumothorax.
Tympany	High	Loud	Musical, drumlike	Normal over stomach. Over lung may indicate tension pneumothorax.

(MCL). At the sixth ICS and left MCL, you'll hear resonance again. As you percuss downward, you'll hear tympany over the gas-filled stomach. If the stomach contains less gas, you'll hear either hyperresonance, resonance, or dullness. On the right side, you should hear resonance, indicating normal lung tissue. Near the fifth to seventh ICS, you'll hear dullness, marking the superior border of the liver.

To percuss the lateral chest, have your patient raise his arms over his head. Percuss laterally, comparing right and left sides as you move downward. These areas should also be resonant.

Diaphragmatic excursion. Next, measure the patient's diaphragmatic excursion. Instruct him to take a deep breath and hold it while you percuss downward on the posterior chest until dullness identifies the lower border of the lung field. Mark

this point. Now ask the patient to exhale and again hold his breath as you percuss upward to the area of dullness. Mark this point, too.

Repeat the procedure on the opposite side of the patient's chest. Then measure the distances between the two marks on each side. Normal diaphragmatic excursion measures about 1½″ to 2½″ (3 to 6 cm), and the diaphragm is slightly higher on the right side.

Abnormal findings. A dull sound over lung areas (which should sound resonant) indicates fluid or solid tissue, such as you might find with pneumonia, atelectasis, pleural effusion, or a tumor. Flatness normally occurs over muscle or bone. If you hear it in the lung, it indicates solid tissue that could stem from atelectasis or, if it's at the lung bases, pleural effusion. Hyperresonance occurs over a fully inflated lung. It's normal in children, but in adults may reflect air trapped in the lungs. That can occur with emphysema, chronic bronchitis, asthma, or pneumothorax. You'd normally expect to hear tympany over the stomach. This sound indicates the presence of gas.

A marked difference in diaphragm level from one side to the other may result from pneumothorax or impaired innervation. Decreased diaphragmatic excursion may be caused by ascites, pregnancy, COPD, atelectasis, pneumonia, pleural effusion, and hepatomegaly.

Auscultating the chest

To assess airflow through your patient's respiratory system, auscultate his lungs and identify normal, abnormal, and adventitious breath sounds (see *Identifying normal and adventitious breath sounds,* page 38). Lung auscultation helps detect abnormal fluid or mucus as well as obstructed passages.

When you're auscultating the patient's chest, instruct him to take full, slow breaths through his mouth. Nose-breathing changes the pitch of lung sounds. Listen for one full inspiration and expiration before moving the stethoscope. If your patient has a lot of hair on his chest, wet and mat it with a damp washcloth to prevent it from causing rubbing sounds that can be confused with crackles.

If your patient tries to accommodate you by breathing quickly and deeply with every movement of the stethoscope, he may hyperventilate. So if he complains he's getting light-headed or dizzy, stop auscultating and allow him to breathe normally for a few minutes.

Posterior chest. Using the diaphragm of your stethoscope, begin auscultating the posterior chest above the scapulae. Then go to the area between the scapulae and the vertebral column. Move laterally beneath the scapulae to the right and left lower lobes. Move the diaphragm methodically, and compare the sounds you hear on both sides of your patient's chest before moving to the next area.

Normally, you'll hear bronchovesicular breath sounds — medium-pitched sounds having the same duration on inspiration and expiration — between the scapulae. You'll hear vesicular breath sounds — soft, low-pitched sounds lasting longer during inspiration — at the lung bases. Decreased or absent breath sounds may result from bronchial obstruction, muscle weakness, obesity, or pleural disease.

Anterior chest. Begin auscultating the anterior chest at the trachea, where you should hear bronchial breath sounds — loud, high-pitched sounds that last longer on expiration. Next, listen for bronchovesicular breath sounds where the mainstem bronchi branch from the trachea, near the second ICS, ¾″ to 1½″ (2 to 4 cm) to either side of the sternum. Using the chest landmarks, listen over the peripheral lung fields for vesicular sounds.

Lateral chest. Be sure to auscultate the lateral chest walls, comparing the right and left sides as you proceed. On the left side, heart sounds diminish breath sounds; on the right side, the liver diminishes them.

Abnormal sounds. Note any normal sounds in an abnormal location, or changes in duration or intensity of normal sounds. Bronchovesicular sounds heard over the peripheral lung areas can indicate a partial

Identifying normal and adventitious breath sounds

Breath sounds are produced by air moving through the tracheobronchoalveolar system. Depending on their location, duration, and intensity, bronchial, bronchovesicular, and vesicular breath sounds may be normal or abnormal. Adventitious breath sounds occur when air passes either through narrowed airways or through moisture, or when the membranes lining the chest cavity and the lungs become inflamed.

Note that the ratios under normal breath sounds indicate the relative durations of each sound during inspiration (I) and expiration (E).

NORMAL BREATH SOUNDS

Type	Location	Ratio	Description
Bronchial	Over the trachea	I / E — 2:3	Loud, high-pitched, and hollow, harsh, or coarse
Broncho-vesicular	Anteriorly, near the main-stem bronchi in the first and second intercostal spaces; posteriorly, between the scapulae	I / E — 1:1	Soft, breezy, and pitched about two notes lower than bronchial sounds
Vesicular	In most of the lungs' peripheral areas (can't be heard over the presternum or scapulae)	I / E — 3:1	Soft, swishy, breezy, and about two notes lower than bronchovesicular sounds

ADVENTITIOUS BREATH SOUNDS

Type	Location	Cause	Description
Crackles	Anywhere; heard in lung bases first with pulmonary edema, usually during inspiratory phase	Air passing through moisture, especially in small airways and alveoli	Light crackling, popping, nonmusical; also classified by pitch: high, medium, or low
Rhonchi	In larger airways, usually during expiratory phase	Fluid or secretions in the large airways or narrowing of large airways	Coarse rattling, usually louder and lower-pitched than crackles; can be described as sonorous, bubbling, moaning, musical, sibilant, and rumbly
Wheezes	Anywhere; occur during inspiration and expiration	Narrowed airways	Creaking, groaning; always high-pitched, musical squeaks
Pleural friction rub	Anterolateral lung field on both inspiration and expiration (with the patient in an upright position)	Inflamed parietal and visceral pleural linings rubbing together	Superficial squeaking or grating

obstruction or decreased aeration. Bronchial sounds heard over the lung areas usually indicate tissue consolidation, such as occurs with pneumonia. They can also result from the turbulence caused by high airway pressures in adult respiratory distress syndrome (ARDS). In a ventilator patient, vesicular breath sounds are louder during inspiration and last longer during expiration, and you'll hear little, if any, pause between inspiration and expiration.

Adventitious sounds. Also note any adventitious breath sounds — sounds that aren't normal in any location. These include crackles, rhonchi, wheezes, and pleural friction rubs. If you hear an adventitious breath sound, record its location and timing in the respiratory cycle — during inspiration, for example.
• *Crackles.* Usually heard on inspiration, crackles indicate intra-alveolar fluid accumulation, atelectasis, or pulmonary fibrosis. You'll also hear them over dependent lung areas in early pulmonary edema.
• *Rhonchi.* You'll hear these bubbly sounds over the larger airways. Usually more pronounced on expiration, they indicate mucus or fluid in the tracheobronchial tree. These sounds are common in smokers, especially in the morning. They often clear when the person coughs.
• *Wheezes.* Heard on inspiration or expiration, wheezes result from air rushing through narrowed passageways in the tracheobronchial tree. The underlying cause can be a mucus plug, bronchospasm, or a tumor.

If you detect crackles, rhonchi, or wheezes, tell your patient to cough and breathe deeply. After letting him rest, listen again to the area where you heard the adventitious sound. Note any changes.
• *Pleural friction rubs.* You'll hear these adventitious sounds on inspiration and expiration. As their name indicates, pleural friction rubs result from the inflamed parietal and visceral pleura rubbing together. Localized rubs are associated with pulmonary infarction; generalized rubs, with pleurisy.

You probably won't hear adventitious breath sounds at all in patients on high-frequency ventilation because of the minute volumes of gas inflating the alveoli and the greatly reduced times for inspiration and expiration — in fact, you may not be able to distinguish the two phases.

Voice sounds. If you've detected any respiratory abnormality during palpation, percussion, or auscultation, assess your patient's voice sounds for vocal fremitus. The significance of vocal fremitus is based on the principle that sound carries best through a solid, not as well through fluid, and poorly through air.

To elicit vocal fremitus, ask your patient to say "99," whisper "one, two, three," and say "ee-ee-ee" while you auscultate his thorax in the systematic way just described. Normally, you should hear vocal fremitus as muffled, unclear sounds, loudest medially and less intense at the lung periphery. Voice sounds that become louder and more distinct are known as bronchophony — an abnormal finding except over the large bronchus. If you hear the words "one, two, three" clearly through your stethoscope, your patient has whispered pectoriloquy, an exaggerated bronchophony. If you hear the sound "ee-ee-ee" as "ay-ay-ay" through the stethoscope, your patient has egophony. You may hear bronchophony, whispered pectoriloquy, and egophony in any patient with consolidated lungs or pleural effusion.

Monitoring oxygen status

Excessive oxygen can be as detrimental as insufficient oxygen. As a result, you have to monitor your patient's arterial oxygen level continuously to ensure that he's getting the best treatment with the fewest complications.

Arterial blood gas (ABG) analysis, continuous $S\bar{v}O_2$ monitoring, and pulse oximetry can help you evaluate your patient's oxygenation, and capnography helps you evaluate his ventilatory status.

ABG analysis

When a patient has respiratory difficulty, ABG analysis is typically the first test ordered by the doctor. It helps evaluate the efficiency of pulmonary gas exchange, assess the integrity of ventilatory control, and determine the blood's acid-base balance. ABG analysis also helps monitor the effectiveness of respiratory therapy.

This test evaluates gas exchange in the lungs by measuring the PaO_2, $PaCO_2$, arterial oxygen saturation (SaO_2), bicarbonate (HCO_3^-) level, and the pH of an arterial blood sample. PaO_2 and SaO_2 indicate how much oxygen the lungs are delivering to the blood; $PaCO_2$ indicates how efficiently the lungs are eliminating carbon dioxide (CO_2). The pH reflects the blood's acid-base level (or the hydrogen ion [H^+] concentration). An acidic pH indicates an H^+ excess; an alkaline pH indicates an H^+ deficit. By evaluating pH, $PaCO_2$, and HCO_3^- in a patient's ar-

terial blood, you can determine his acid-base balance.

To get the most accurate results from ABG analysis, wait at least 15 to 20 minutes after an intermittent positive-pressure breathing (IPPB) treatment, suctioning, or a change in respiratory therapy or ventilator settings.

Obtaining blood samples. A percutaneous blood sample for ABG analysis can be drawn from the radial, brachial, or femoral artery. Most hospitals permit only doctors to perform femoral artery punctures, so check your hospital's policy before proceeding.

The preferred site is the radial artery. Before using it, though, you must perform Allen's test to ensure that the ulnar artery can adequately perfuse the patient's hand should the radial artery be damaged (see *How to perform Allen's test*).

Radial artery puncture. You'll first need to collect the necessary equipment. Many hospitals have commercially prepared kits that contain these items: a 10-ml glass or plastic leur-lock syringe made especially for drawing blood gases, a 1-ml ampule of aqueous heparin (1:1,000), a 1½" 20G needle, a 1" 22G needle, a povidone-iodine sponge, an alcohol sponge, two 2" × 2" gauze pads, a rubber cap for syringe hub or a rubber stopper for needle, a plastic bag to fill with ice, a label, and an adhesive bandage. You'll also need clean gloves, a towel, and some ice. When you have this equipment, follow these steps:
• Heparinize the syringe. Eject all but about 0.1 ml of the heparin through the needle. If you don't heparinize the syringe or if you leave too much heparin in it, the test results may be inaccurate.

How to perform Allen's test

Before performing a radial artery puncture, use Allen's test to determine if the ulnar artery can supply the hand with enough blood should the radial artery become damaged. Rest the patient's arm on the bedside stand, supporting the wrist with a rolled towel; don't hyperextend the wrist. Ask him to clench his fist. With your index and middle fingers, exert pressure on the radial and ulnar arteries.

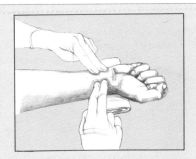

Hold this position for a few seconds. While applying pressure to both arteries, ask your patient to unclench and relax his hand. The palm will be blanched because you've occluded blood flow to the area.

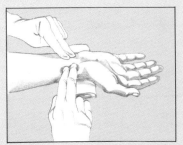

Now, release the pressure on the ulnar artery. If the hand becomes flushed, indicating a rush of oxygenated blood to the area, you can safely proceed with the radial artery puncture.

If the hand remains blanched, repeat the test on the other arm. If neither arm produces a positive result, use the brachial artery for arterial puncture.

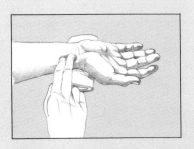

- Remove the needle from the syringe and replace it with the other needle for the puncture.
- Place the rolled towel under your patient's wrist for support.
- Palpate to locate the artery.
- Put on clean gloves before puncturing the artery to protect yourself against blood-borne infection. Re-

member, gloves can protect only as long as they're intact. If they're punctured, replace them.
- Clean the puncture site with a povidine-iodine sponge, wiping in a circular motion starting from the center and spiraling outward.
- Allow the area to dry and clean it in the same way with an alcohol

sponge. Again allow the skin to dry.
• Palpate again to locate the artery.
• Hold the needle, bevel facing upward, at a 45-degree angle over the radial artery. Tell the patient he may feel a burning or throbbing sensation for a few seconds.
• Puncture the skin and the arterial wall in one motion, following the path of the artery. Be careful not to apply too much pressure. You may go right through the far wall of the artery and cause a hematoma or even nick the periosteum of the bone, causing the patient severe pain.
• Watch for blood backflow in the syringe. Don't pull back on the plunger because arterial blood should enter the syringe automatically. If it doesn't, the needle may be in a vein — not the radial artery. Determining whether the needle is in the artery can be difficult, particularly if the patient is hypotensive (blood may not pulse into the syringe because of low pressure) or hypoxemic (poor arterial oxygenation can cause very dark blood resembling venous blood).
• Fill the syringe to the 5-ml mark.

After collecting the sample, press a gauze pad firmly over the puncture site for at least 5 minutes or until the bleeding stops. If your patient is receiving anticoagulant therapy, apply pressure for 10 to 15 minutes. You may need to ask a co-worker to hold the gauze pad in place while you prepare the sample for transport to the laboratory. Don't ask the patient to hold the pad. If insufficient pressure is applied, a large, painful hematoma may form, which would prevent the site from being used for future arterial punctures. When the bleeding stops, apply a small adhesive bandage to the site.

Check the syringe for air bubbles, which can alter PaO_2 results, by holding the syringe upright and gently tapping it on the side. If you see air bubbles, remove them by holding the syringe upright and slowly ejecting some of the blood with the air bubbles onto a gauze pad. Insert the needle into a rubber stopper, or remove the needle and place a rubber cap directly on the syringe hub. This prevents the sample from leaking and keeps air out of the syringe.

Label the syringe and place it in an ice-filled plastic bag. Attach a properly completed laboratory request slip, and send the sample to the laboratory immediately. The laboratory slip should include the following information: whether the patient was breathing room air or receiving oxygen; the amount of oxygen he was receiving; the type of oxygen delivery device; the patient's position, rectal temperature, and respiratory rate; and, if he's on a ventilator, the fraction of inspired oxygen (FIO_2), tidal volume, rate, mode, and PEEP.

Brachial artery puncture. To perform a brachial artery puncture, you'd follow the same steps as above. The only difference is that you'd hold the needle at a 60-degree angle when puncturing the artery.

Arterial line. You may also draw an ABG specimen from an arterial line. To do so, prepare the syringe as described above. Then proceed as follows:
• Turn the stopcock handle toward the syringe port and activate the fast-flush release of the continuous flush device. This will flush the arterial line.
• Unscrew the stopcock cap, and attach an unheparinized 10-ml syringe.
• Turn the stopcock handle back toward the continuous flush device

to initiate arterial blood flow.
• Aspirate 5 ml of blood by pulling back gently on the plunger.
• Turn the stopcock handle toward the syringe port to shut off arterial blood flow. Then remove and discard the syringe.
• Secure the heparinized syringe to the syringe port. Make sure the syringe is free of air bubbles, which could alter test results.
• Turn the stopcock handle back toward the continuous flush device to initiate arterial blood flow.
• Withdraw between 3 and 5 ml of blood.
• Turn the stopcock handle straight up again and remove the syringe.
• Hold the barrel and plunger of the syringe securely to avoid spilling the sample.
• Check the syringe for air bubbles, as described above.
• Place the rubber cap on the syringe, and put it in the ice-filled plastic bag. Label the bag as described above and send it to the laboratory immediately.
• Place a 2″ × 2″ gauze pad over the syringe port. Turn the stopcock handle toward the patient. Then activate the fast-flush release of the continuous flush device to allow I.V. solution to clear the blood from the syringe port.
• Replace the cap on the syringe port. Then turn the stopcock handle so that it points straight up. Activate the fast-flush release again to flush the arterial line completely.

Evaluating the results. The normal ABG values are as follows:
• pH: 7.35 to 7.45
• PaO_2: 75 to 100 mm Hg (decreases with age)
• $PaCO_2$: 35 to 45 mm Hg
• HCO_3^-: 22 to 26 mEq/liter
• SaO_2: 95% to 100%.
By analyzing the patient's ABG

results, you can evaluate his acid-base balance and oxygenation.
• *Acid-base balance.* To determine your patient's acid-base balance, first look at his pH. Remember, a high pH means a low concentration of H^+, indicating alkalinity; a low pH means a high concentration of H^+, indicating acidity.

$PaCO_2$ reflects alveolar ventilation. A high $PaCO_2$, which indicates acidity, means that CO_2 is being retained by the lungs through hypoventilation. A low $PaCO_2$ indicates alkalinity. A patient with such a reading is hyperventilating, or blowing off CO_2.

HCO_3^- reflects the renally regulated or metabolic component of the body's acid-base balance. A low HCO_3^- indicates metabolic acidosis; a high HCO_3^-, metabolic alkalosis.

If your patient's pH is acidotic, determine the cause. Check to see if his $PaCO_2$ is higher than 45 mm Hg or if his HCO_3^- is lower than 22 mEq/liter. Because CO_2 is eliminated by the lungs, you know that a low pH with an abnormal buildup of $PaCO_2$ means respiratory acidosis. And because HCO_3^- concentration is produced by the renal system, you probably also know that a low pH with a low HCO_3^- means metabolic acidosis.

In the same way, you can determine the cause if your patient's pH is alkalotic. Check to see if his $PaCO_2$ is less than 35 mm Hg or his HCO_3^- is greater than 26 mEq/liter. A decrease in $PaCO_2$ combined with a high pH spells respiratory alkalosis. A high HCO_3^- combined with a high pH signifies metabolic alkalosis.

If your patient's pH falls within normal limits but is close to abnormal, you should note whether it's borderline high or borderline low. A pH that's borderline low, combined with a high $PaCO_2$, indicates compensated respiratory acidosis. The patient's lungs can't eliminate enough CO_2, but his kidneys are compensating by retaining HCO_3^-. In contrast, if the pH is borderline high and the HCO_3^- and $PaCO_2$ are low, your patient has compensated metabolic acidosis.

• *Oxygenation.* After you've evaluated your patient's acid-base balance, you must assess his oxygenation. The PaO_2 measures this, but you also need to know the FIO_2 the patient was receiving when you drew the blood sample. The normal PaO_2 range of 75 to 100 mm Hg applies to a person breathing room air. (The normal values are lower in elderly people and neonates because of decreased lung compliance.) An increase in FIO_2 should produce an increase in PaO_2. If it doesn't, try to determine why. A below-normal PaO_2 can be caused by airway obstruction, inspiration of oxygen-poor air, respiratory muscle weakness, inhibition of the respiratory center, or a ventilation-perfusion mismatch.

SaO_2 is a measure of the amount of hemoglobin that's saturated by oxygen compared to the total amount of oxygen that the hemoglobin could carry. The oxygen that's combined with hemoglobin is kept in reserve to replenish the plasma when oxygen is used to meet metabolic demands. Normally, 95% to 100% oxygen saturation is needed to replenish the plasma. Decreased saturation results from decreased oxygen supply and increased oxygen demand.

Continuous $S\bar{v}O_2$ monitoring

Mixed venous oxygen saturation ($S\bar{v}O_2$) reflects venous oxygen returned to the heart and indicates perfusion adequacy. The normal

$S\bar{v}O_2$ ranges between 70% and 75%. By monitoring $S\bar{v}O_2$, you can assess how completely body tissue uses oxygen. (See *How the body balances oxygen supply and demand.*)

A special pulmonary artery catheter with light-emitting and light-receiving fiber optics allows you to monitor $S\bar{v}O_2$ continuously. This catheter is attached to an optical module that's connected to a microprocessor-based monitor (see *Understanding the fiber-optic $S\bar{v}O_2$ monitor,* page 46). Some $S\bar{v}O_2$ devices can also monitor cardiac output and I.V. titration rates.

This type of monitoring does have a disadvantage: It's an invasive procedure. Thus, the risk of infection increases in patients who are already susceptible.

Indications. $S\bar{v}O_2$ monitoring can be used to facilitate rapid assessment and intervention in a hemodynamically unstable patient who becomes hypoxic or hypoxemic. You may also use $S\bar{v}O_2$ monitoring to quickly assess your patient's response to drug administration, suctioning, or ventilator setting changes — including changes in FIO_2 and PEEP. And you may monitor a critically ill patient — particularly if he has severe respiratory insufficiency or he's recovering from cardiothoracic surgery.

Setting up the monitor. First, connect the optical module to the computer and turn the system on. Verify that the time and date on the screen are correct. Then, make sure the computer is in the correct operating mode, and set the low and high oxygen saturation alarm limits — usually to 10% above and 10% below the patient's baseline. Calibrate the machine according to the manufacturer's instructions be-

How the body balances oxygen supply and demand

The balance between oxygen supply and demand depends on cardiac output, arterial oxygen saturation (SaO_2), and hemoglobin (Hb) on one side of the scale, and tissue oxygen consumption on the other. Cardiac output is the volume of blood pumped from the heart each minute. A normal cardiac output, 4 to 8 liters/minute, is maintained by a normal heart rate and stroke volume. SaO_2, expressed as a percentage, represents the amount of oxygen bound to Hb divided by the amount of oxygen that could bind to Hb. Normal SaO_2 is 95% to 100%.

Keep in mind, however, that if the person doesn't have a normal Hb level — 14 to 18 g/dl (140 to 180 g/liter) for men and 11.5 to 15.5 g/dl (115 to 155 g/liter) for women — tissue oxygenation may be low even if SaO_2 is normal.

Tissue oxygen consumption refers to the amount of oxygen used by the tissue per minute; normally, this is 240 to 250 ml/minute. Mixed venous oxygen saturation ($S\bar{v}O_2$) measures tissue oxygen consumption. Normal $S\bar{v}O_2$ is 70% to 75%. The lists below show some common causes of increased and decreased $S\bar{v}O_2$.

INCREASED $S\bar{v}O_2$	DECREASED $S\bar{v}O_2$
• Increased cardiac output	• Decreased cardiac output
• Increased SaO_2	• Decreased SaO_2
• Vasoconstriction	• Vasodilation
• Septic shock	• Cardiogenic shock
• Hypothermia	• Hyperthermia or fever
• Anesthesia	• Shivering
• Sedation	• Seizures
• Chemical paralysis	• Positive end-expiratory pressure
	• High airway pressure

fore attaching it to the catheter's optical connector. Such preinsertion calibration will be more accurate than in vivo calibration. Plus, you'll start receiving accurate readings as soon as the optical module is connected.

Next, insert the catheter's optical connector into the optical module. To avoid the need to recalibrate, make sure the catheter remains connected to the optical module whenever the patient is transported for a procedure or test. Perform an in vivo calibration daily (you lose the accuracy of the preinsertion calibration when you do this, but the laboratory will verify your results when you send in the blood sample). Also, do such calibrations if

the catheter does become disconnected or if the $S\bar{v}O_2$ reading given by the computer differs from that of a pulmonary artery blood sample checked by the laboratory.

To perform an in vivo calibration, set the computer on the blood-drawing mode. Obtain a blood sample from the distal lumen of the pulmonary artery catheter, place it in ice, and send it to the laboratory for oxygen saturation analysis. Then enter the saturation percentage in the computer.

Evaluating monitor readings. The monitor gives continuous readings, but how often you record them will depend on your patient's status. You may routinely document them

EQUIPMENT

Understanding the fiber-optic $S\bar{v}O_2$ monitor

With this monitor, which is connected to a special pulmonary artery catheter, you can continuously check your patient's mixed venous oxygen saturation ($S\bar{v}O_2$).

Readings are obtained when light from one optical fiber is emitted from the tip of the catheter, then reflected by oxygen-saturated hemoglobin (oxyhemoglobin) and returned by the light-receiving optical fiber to a photodetector in the optical module. The light signal is converted into an electrical signal, the $S\bar{v}O_2$ is averaged, and the percentage of oxyhemoglobin saturation is displayed digitally.

Updated $S\bar{v}O_2$ values are displayed every second. This allows rapid assessment and intervention before the patient suffers any significant tissue deoxygenation.

Besides the numerical reading, the screen displays a graph of changes in $S\bar{v}O_2$.

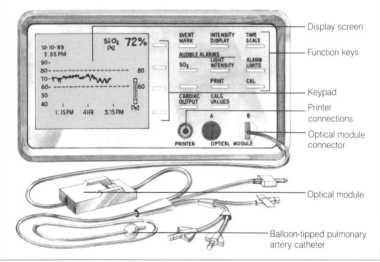

only once an hour. But you should also note any changes after the patient receives a treatment or performs an activity.

Expect to see decreased $S\bar{v}O_2$ after intubation or suctioning and when your patient is turned or weighed. All of these activities involve increased muscle movement that results in decreased gas exchange or increased metabolic demands for oxygen. PEEP therapy can also cause $S\bar{v}O_2$ to drop by in-

creasing airway and alveolar pressure, which decreases cardiac output. But you may also see an increase after the start of PEEP therapy because arterial oxygenation will improve. You'll see an increase in $S\bar{v}O_2$ after the start of drug therapy, such as dobutamine or amrinone infusions, because such therapy results in improved cardiac output and tissue perfusion (see *Understanding $S\bar{v}O_2$ waveform variations*).

If you see an unexpected decrease in S$\bar{v}O_2$, you'll need to assess to determine the cause. Check first for adequate oxygenation. If your patient is on a ventilator, see if the settings have been changed. Is the machine delivering the proper FIO$_2$ and tidal volume? If he's being weaned from the ventilator, a decrease in S$\bar{v}O_2$ may mean that he's tolerating the weaning poorly and needs to be put back on the ventilator. If you find no problems with oxygenation, check for evidence of decreased cardiac output.

If you note an unexpected increase in S$\bar{v}O_2$, check for evidence of decreased oxygen use in the tissues. This may result from shock, left-to-right shunting, or hypothermia, for example. If your patient is on a ventilator, check to see if the FIO$_2$ setting has been increased.

Troubleshooting. If you find no physical causes for unexpected S$\bar{v}O_2$ variations, troubleshoot the machine to see if the problem is mechanical. Several factors can adversely affect the machine's ability to provide accurate readings. Fibers in the plastic fiber-optic tip can be easily crushed, causing a reduction in or a loss of the signal. If the catheter is left in place for more than 48 hours, a small thrombus may form on its tip, producing inaccurate readings.

Consider, too, that false information may have been programmed into the computer. Or the catheter may be improperly positioned so that it wedges in the pulmonary artery, falsely increasing the S$\bar{v}O_2$ reading. Another possibility: A kinked catheter may produce a falsely decreased reading.

Pulse oximetry

This procedure allows you to moni-

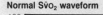

Understanding S$\bar{v}O_2$ waveform variations

The first illustration is a normal S$\bar{v}O_2$ waveform. The second depicts variations you can expect to see when a patient is suctioned, turned, and weighed. And the third shows you the variations produced when positive end-expiratory pressure (PEEP) is initiated and FIO$_2$ is decreased.

Normal S$\bar{v}O_2$ waveform

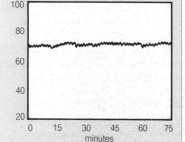

S$\bar{v}O_2$ with patient activities

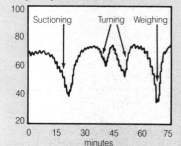

S$\bar{v}O_2$ with PEEP and FIO$_2$ changes

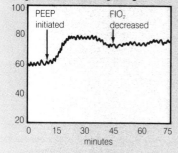

tor a patient's SaO_2 noninvasively. Fairly simple to learn, pulse oximetry is painless, accurate, cost-effective, and easy to use. This procedure also provides immediate and continuous results.

However, pulse oximetry doesn't provide all the information you need to thoroughly evaluate your patient's ventilatory status. So you still need to perform routine ABG analysis.

Pulse oximeters measure the absorption (or amplitude) of wavelengths of light passing through parts of the body that are highly perfused by arterial blood (see *How pulse oximetry works*). Because saturated and reduced hemoglobin absorb different wavelengths, the computer can calculate the SaO_2, which is then displayed on a monitor. Some units can also provide a printout of the resulting waveforms and numeric values for a permanent record.

Though false readings are rare, certain factors may affect the accuracy of the SaO_2 measurements. For example, dyes used in cardiac output studies and high levels of carboxyhemoglobin in patients who smoke will produce falsely elevated readings. And you'll get falsely low readings if your patient has high serum bilirubin levels or poor perfusion.

Indications. As an adjunct to physical assessment, pulse oximetry is used for continuous assessment of oxygenation status in critical care units, operating rooms, recovery rooms, and emergency departments. The test also helps you assess oxygenation status during diagnostic testing and outpatient follow-up. During general anesthesia and immediate post-anesthesia recovery, continuous evaluation of SaO_2 per-

mits early intervention before hypoxia or other potential complications develop.

In patients with acute problems, such as cardiac or respiratory failure, COPD, interstitial lung disease, pulmonary emboli, drug overdose, hemorrhage, or head trauma, you can use pulse oximetry to monitor SaO_2 trends. This helps you evaluate the progression of the underlying problem and the effectiveness of treatments such as oxygen therapy and mechanical ventilation.

You can also monitor SaO_2 trends to help evaluate the hypoxic effect of suctioning, postural drainage, and normal activities of daily living in patients with chronic lung disease or sleep apnea. Or you may need to monitor these trends in patients undergoing diagnostic procedures, such as exercise testing, cardiac catheterization, bronchoscopy, bronchography, or ventilation-perfusion scans.

Setting up the equipment. Follow the manufacturer's instructions for the unit you're using. Attach the power cord, and select the probe you're going to use.
• *Placing the probe.* If you're using an ear probe, massage your patient's earlobe with an alcohol sponge for 10 to 20 seconds until mild erythema indicates adequate vascularization. Then attach the probe to the patient's earlobe or pinna, according to the instructions. Maintaining good contact on the ear may be difficult, but it's important. If the probe slips, the low-perfusion alarm will go off. For prolonged monitoring or exercise testing, use an ear probe stabilizer, if one comes with the unit.

A finger probe is usually the best choice for adults because it gives slightly more accurate readings than the ear probe. However, both usually provide readings that fall within an acceptably reliable range.

Place the probe on the patient's index finger, unless he's obese. If he is, select a smaller finger. If the patient has long nails, you may position the probe on the sides of the finger, depending on the type of probe. And be sure to remove any nail polish or false fingernails. Place the probe over the patient's finger so that the light beams and light sensors oppose each other.

A nasal probe, applied over the nasal bridge, allows you to make oximetric readings even when your patient has extremely low perfusion. Pulsation of the nasal septal anterior ethmoid artery, supplied by the internal carotid artery, can be sensed long after the finger pulse disappears. Keep in mind, however, that this probe can be used only on immobile, anesthetized, or paralyzed patients because it's highly sensitive to movement and respirations. The probe proves especially helpful during surgery, when other sites can't be used because of severe vasoconstriction.

With neonates and infants, you can wrap a probe around the foot so that light beams and light sensors oppose each other. This site is preferred because infants usually move their feet less than their hands. For larger infants, you can use a probe that fits on the great toe. Protect the probe by putting a sock on the baby's foot. If the foot isn't accessible, you can wrap the probe around the palm of the baby's hand.

• *Setting up the device.* Now connect the probe to the monitor box and turn on the power switch. After a few seconds, a saturation reading and pulse waveform will appear on the screen. If the device is work-

How pulse oximetry works

Light-emitting diodes in the transducer send red and infrared light beams through tissues. A light-sensitive photodetector – the sensor – opposite the transducer measures the transmitted light as it passes through the vascular bed, records the relative amount of color absorbed by arterial blood, and transmits the data to a monitor, which displays the information with each heartbeat. If the SaO_2 level or pulse rate exceeds or drops below preset limits, it activates visual and audible alarms.

Finger transducer

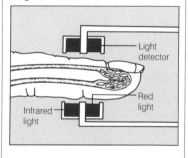

ing properly, you'll hear a beep and see the display light and the pulse searchlight flash. The SaO_2 and pulse rate displays should show stationary zeros. After four to six heartbeats, these displays will start showing information with each beat, and the pulse amplitude indicator will begin tracking the pulse. You'll also hear a beep rising in pitch as SaO_2 increases and falling as SaO_2 decreases with each beat.

Set the high and low SaO_2 alarm limits and the high and low pulse alarm limits. On some devices, certain limits are preset but can be adjusted according to hospital policy, patient condition, or doctor's order. The high SaO_2 will be preset at 100% for adults and 95% for neonates; low SaO_2 will be 85% for adults and 80% for neonates. Pulse settings also differ by age: High pulse rate is preset at 140 beats/minute for adults and 200 beats/minute for neonates; low pulse rate is 55 beats/minute for adults and 100 beats/minute for neonates. If the alarm volume is turned off or down, turn it up.

With some units, you can select an averaging mode that lets readings take place at 3- to 6-second intervals. The three modes are:
• short — for sleep and special studies with inactive patients
• moderate — for relatively inactive patients
• long — for active patients (used during stress testing and for continuous monitoring of small children).

Evaluating the readings. Although the normal SaO_2 is considered 95% to 100% (slightly lower for neonates more than 1 hour old), a particular patient's normal value may vary — especially if he has underlying chronic pulmonary disease. So when you begin testing a patient with pulse oximetry, you need to establish a baseline. Confirm the accuracy of the readings, using ABG analysis. Then monitor the oximetry readings and note any changes.

If you note a decrease in SaO_2, assess the patient's status to determine if intervention is necessary. As with $S\bar{v}O_2$ monitoring, values will decrease after some treatments, such as suctioning, and with activity, even moving about in bed. If the decrease doesn't result from such causes, rule out any conditions that could decrease arterial oxygenation. Auscultate the patient's lungs for adventitious breath sounds that can indicate fluid or consolidation, which would interfere with oxygen-

ation. If the patient is receiving mechanical ventilation, make sure the problem isn't with the ventilator. You may need additional ABG analysis to determine the underlying cause of the change in SaO_2.

Increasing values usually indicate improvement in oxygenation — either from improvement in the underlying condition or an increase in inspired oxygen. If the patient's SaO_2 remains above normal, however, you should reevaluate his respiratory support. Prolonged exposure to high levels of oxygen can cause oxygen toxicity and eventual fibrosis of pulmonary tissue. Monitoring SaO_2 allows you to reduce the amount of inspired oxygen quickly and still maintain adequate oxygenation.

Special considerations. When the SaO_2 or pulse rate falls outside the alarm limits, the corresponding indicator light and SaO_2 display on the front panel flash and the alarm sounds steadily. Loss of the pulse signal or transducer connection also makes the alarm sound. In this case, however, the SaO_2 and pulse rate displays go blank, and the pulse search indicator flashes.

Frequently check circulation to the probe site. To prevent skin breakdown, remove the probe every 2 hours. Inspect the skin under the probe for irritation at least once a day.

When you no longer need the probe, remove it, turn off the power, and unplug the power cord. Clean the probe by rubbing it gently with a manufacturer-recommended cleaner, usually alcohol, bleach, or glutaraldehyde (Cidex). Don't immerse it. If your patient has been in isolation, sterilize the entire unit in ethylene oxide or follow the manufacturer's recommendations.

Understanding the capnometer

A capnometer measures end-tidal CO_2 in exhaled air. Values are displayed numerically and graphically to aid a continuous assessment of cardiovascular and respiratory status.

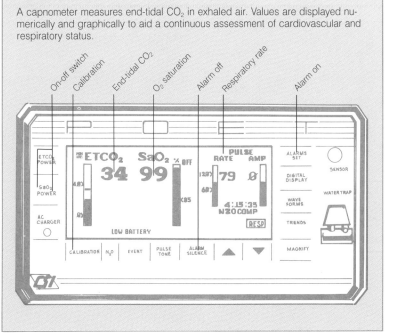

Capnography

Capnometers monitor CO_2 levels, usually by measuring the partial pressure of end-tidal CO_2 ($ETCO_2$) in expired air. Most capnometers use infrared absorption spectroscopy. Of the common gases in exhaled air, only CO_2 and water vapor absorb infrared light. And the capnometer evaporates the water vapor by dehumidifying the gas sample.

Capnometers display CO_2 values in one of three ways: as a percentage (%), in millimeters of mercury (mm Hg), or in kilopascals (kPa). The monitor also displays CO_2 values graphically as a continuous waveform, or capnogram (see *Understanding the capnometer*).

Capnography allows you to measure ventilation, perfusion, and metabolism noninvasively. Used mostly in the operating room by anesthesiologists, capnography may also be used for patients being mechanically ventilated, weaned from a mechanical ventilator, or resuscitated by cardiopulmonary resuscitation (CPR) in the intensive care unit or emergency department.

Indications. Specific indications for capnography include the following:
• *To determine placement of an endotracheal tube in the operating room.* If esophageal intubation occurs, CO_2 may be expelled during ventilation of the stomach. The

resulting capnogram looks very different from a normal tracheal capnogram. You'll note a reduction in CO_2 concentration with each successive gastric ventilation. This rapid decrease is consistent with the predictable washout of CO_2 from the stomach.

• *To detect apnea.* If the capnometer doesn't detect CO_2 or if the CO_2 reading drops to zero, the apnea alarm will sound, indicating that the patient's lungs aren't being ventilated. Such apnea may result from many factors, including disconnection of the endotracheal tube from the anesthesia delivery system or ventilator, ventilator malfunction, or loss of gas supply pressure or electricity. The apnea alarm may also be triggered by disconnection of the CO_2 sensor or gas sampling line or failure of the capnometer itself.

• *To detect early signs of shock or pulmonary embolus.* You may use capnography to monitor critically ill patients for shock or pulmonary embolus. A gradual fall in $ETCO_2$ could indicate increased dead-air space (wasted ventilation) from decreased lung perfusion.

• *To decrease the frequency of ABG measurements.* Used with pulse oximetry, capnography may decrease the need for ABG analysis when you're monitoring a critically ill patient. Capnography alone can decrease the need for ABG analysis in a patient being weaned from mechanical ventilation.

• *To assess the efficacy of CPR.* During cardiac arrest and CPR, CO_2 accumulates in mixed venous blood. Excretion of CO_2 through the lungs during CPR is believed to depend primarily on cardiac output and lung perfusion. So the $ETCO_2$ level may be a noninvasive indicator of both.

You won't see capnography used for a patient on high-frequency ventilation, even for one of these indications. End-tidal gas in these patients consists mostly of gas from conducting airways, not from the alveoli. And entrainment mixes expired gas with room air, making capnography useless.

Setting up a capnometer. Begin by calibrating the capnometer according to the manufacturer's instructions. Then attach the power cord to the receptacle on the monitor. After making sure the sample tube assembly is in good condition, connect one end to the sample inlet connector. You'll connect the other end when you're ready to use the monitor.

The capnograph has both audible and visual alarms that will alert you to a CO_2 value above or below the limits you set. The monitor also has alarms to warn of monitor failure and, as mentioned, apnea. Be sure to set these controls as ordered, following the manufacturer's instructions.

Evaluating capnograms. At 760 mm Hg of atmospheric pressure (95% concentration), a normal CO_2 reading is 38 mm Hg. In patients with normal perfusion and ventilation, CO_2 measurements closely reflect $PaCO_2$.

A capnogram displays changes in CO_2 concentration during the entire respiratory cycle. The shape of the waveform that follows a mechanical breath in a patient with normal lungs differs little from that of a spontaneous breath. You'll analyze waveforms for five characteristics:

• height — depends on the $ETCO_2$ value
• frequency — depends on the respiratory rate

• rhythm — depends on the state of the patient's respiratory center or the function of the ventilator

• baseline — should be at the zero level

• shape — only one shape is normal. (See *Interpreting capnograms,* page 54.)

Normal capnogram. On the capnogram, each respiratory cycle is divided into four phases: inspiratory baseline, expiratory upstroke, expiratory plateau, and inspiratory downstroke.

The *inspiratory baseline* is recorded as fresh gas passes through the CO_2 sampling site and moves toward the patient's lungs. The CO_2 tension measured during this phase should be zero.

The *expiratory upstroke* begins as alveolar gas containing CO_2 reaches the sampling site. The expired CO_2 concentration rises quickly as alveolar gas replaces the inspiratory gas in the anatomic dead space.

The *expiratory plateau* represents exhalation of alveolar gas. The line should be horizontal and smooth, even in a patient receiving mechanical ventilation.

The *inspiratory downstroke* should be steep. When inspiration begins, fresh gas quickly washes away any CO_2 remaining from the previous exhalation, so the volume of gas at the sampling site is small.

Abnormal capnogram. You may see abnormal variations in each phase, depending on the cause. For example, a prolonged expiratory upstroke may result from slow exhalation, uneven emptying of the alveoli, a partially obstructed endotracheal tube, COPD, or bronchospasm. Irregular expiratory plateaus may stem from such problems as displacement of the endotracheal tube.

Be aware that high levels of oxygen, nitrous oxide, water vapor, and halogenated anesthetic vapors in exhaled air may interfere with the results. Many units can automatically adjust the reading when high-flow oxygen or nitrous oxide is used. Still, ABG analysis should be used when you need precise $PaCO_2$ measurements.

Verifying findings. You can interpret the capnogram most accurately by comparing it with other findings recorded simultaneously. These findings include:

• ECG and heart rate
• blood pressure
• body temperature
• $PaCO_2$
• PaO_2
• airway pressure
• central venous pressure
• acid-base status
• respiratory rate
• breathing pattern.

You should also correlate capnometry readings with signs and symptoms of hypercapnia. In a patient who's awake, increasing confusion and behavioral changes may indicate an elevated $PaCO_2$. Other signs and symptoms of hypercapnia include flushed skin, muscle twitching, and headache. Remember, in early stages of hypercapnia, blood pressure will be elevated; in later stages, it'll fall to hypotensive levels.

Pulmonary function tests

Pulmonary function tests (PFTs) measure the lungs' capacity and their ability to transfer gases. These tests help to distinguish between obstructive and restrictive lung diseases, help establish a baseline for evaluating the progression of

Interpreting capnograms

On a capnogram, each respiratory cycle is divided into four phases: inspiratory baseline, expiratory upstroke, expiratory plateau, and inspiratory downstroke.

Normal capnogram. The letters below indicate the phases of a normal respiratory cycle:
- E: inspiratory baseline (beginning of exhalation)
- E-F: anatomic dead-space gas being exhaled
- F-G: ascending portion of waveform, reflecting expiratory upstroke (increasing concentration of CO_2 from increasingly distal airways)
- G-H: alveolar plateau, reflecting expiratory plateau (containing mixed alveolar gases)
- H: end-tidal CO_2
- H-I: descending portion of waveform, reflecting inspiratory downstroke (inspiratory phase showing rapidly decreasing CO_2 concentration as fresh gas is inhaled)
- J: end of inspiratory phase; airways contain fresh gas.

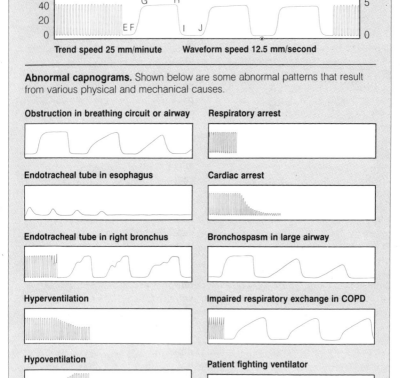

Abnormal capnograms. Shown below are some abnormal patterns that result from various physical and mechanical causes.

Obstruction in breathing circuit or airway

Respiratory arrest

Endotracheal tube in esophagus

Cardiac arrest

Endotracheal tube in right bronchus

Bronchospasm in large airway

Hyperventilation

Impaired respiratory exchange in COPD

Hypoventilation

Patient fighting ventilator

a disease or a response to treatment, and, when performed during exercise, can determine how much exertion a patient can tolerate before experiencing dyspnea.

Complete pulmonary function testing is usually done in the pulmonary function laboratory, where several different techniques may be used, such as spirometry, nitrogen washout, helium dilution, carbon monoxide diffusion, radionuclide perfusion imaging, pneumotachometry, and plethysmography. Many of these tests aren't routinely performed, however, because the equipment isn't available in all institutions.

Direct and indirect tests

Most PFT results are obtained by using a spirometer to measure certain lung volumes, then calculating other measurements from predetermined formulas (see *Interpreting pulmonary function tests,* pages 56 to 58). Of the tests used to determine lung volume, tidal volume (VT) and expiratory reserve volume (ERV) are direct spirographic measurements; minute volume (MV), inspiratory reserve volume (IRV), and residual volume (RV) are calculated from the results of other PFTs (see *Reading a spirogram,* page 59).

Of the tests used to measure lung capacity, vital capacity (VC), inspiratory capacity (IC), functional residual capacity (FRC), and peak expiratory flow (PEF) may be measured directly or calculated from the results of other tests. Forced vital capacity (FVC), flow-volume curve, forced expiratory volume (FEV), and maximal voluntary ventilation (MVV) are direct spirographic measurements. Total lung capacity (TLC) and forced expiratory flow ($FEF_{25\%-75\%}$) are calculated from the results of other tests.

Although a complete pulmonary function study helps determine the patient's exact diagnosis, bedside tests are extremely helpful in monitoring disease progression, assessing the patient's ability to cough effectively, evaluating his response to treatment, verifying the accuracy of respiratory support equipment, and evaluating his readiness for and response to weaning.

Bedside tests. Equipment you'll use for bedside testing includes spirometers, flowmeters, and pressure manometers. Among bedside tests commonly ordered are tests for tidal volume, minute volume, vital capacity, maximum inspiratory pressure, inspiratory capacity, forced vital capacity, forced expiratory volume, forced expiratory flow, and peak expiratory flow.

With a mechanically ventilated patient, you may need to measure peak and plateau pressures. (Some clinicians don't consider these measures of pulmonary function to be PFTs.) These pressures can determine the effective and static compliances of the lungs. Some ventilators can monitor peak and plateau pressures continuously.

To assess whether a patient can be weaned, you can measure vital capacity, forced expiratory volume in 1 second (FEV_1), and minute volume. Maximum inspiratory pressure gives you an indication of his muscle strength and maximum voluntary ventilation, an indication of his endurance. You may also measure the inspiratory peak, plateau, and end-expiratory pressure to determine his lung compliance.

Tidal volume
You can measure tidal volume at the bedside with a Wright spirometer.

(Text continues on page 58.)

Interpreting pulmonary function tests

MEASUREMENT OF PULMONARY FUNCTION	METHOD OF CALCULATION	IMPLICATIONS
Tidal volume (VT): amount of air inhaled or exhaled during normal breathing	Determine the spirographic measurement for 10 breaths, and then divide by 10.	Decreased VT may indicate restrictive disease and requires further testing, such as full pulmonary function studies or chest radiography.
Minute volume (MV): total amount of air breathed per minute	Multiply VT by the respiratory rate.	Normal MV can occur in emphysema. Decreased MV may indicate other diseases, such as pulmonary edema. Increased MV can occur with acidosis, increased CO_2, decreased PaO_2, and exercise.
Maximum inspiratory pressure (MIP): the amount of pressure generated when attempting to initiate an inhalation	Measure using inspiratory pressure manometer.	Decreased MIP appears in neuromuscular disorders and indicates need to initiate mechanical ventilation. Improvement can help determine successful weaning.
Inspiratory reserve volume (IRV): amount of air inspired in excess of normal inspiration	Subtract VT from inspiratory capacity.	Abnormal IRV alone doesn't indicate respiratory dysfunction; IRV decreases during normal exercise.
Expiratory reserve volume (ERV): amount of air that can be forcibly exhaled beyond VT.	Use direct spirographic measurement.	ERV varies, even in healthy persons, but usually decreases in the obese.
Residual volume (RV): amount of air remaining in the lungs after forced expiration	Subtract ERV from functional residual capacity.	RV greater than 35% of total lung capacity after maximal expiratory effort may indicate obstructive disease.
Vital capacity (VC): total volume of air that can be exhaled after maximum inspiration	Use direct spirographic measurement, or add VT, IRV, and ERV.	Normal or increased VC with decreased flow rates may indicate any condition that causes a reduction in functional pulmonary tissue, such as pulmonary edema. Decreased VC with normal or increased flow rates may indicate decreased respiratory effort resulting from neuromuscular disease, drug overdose, or head injury; decreased thoracic expansion; or limited movement of diaphragm.
Inspiratory capacity (IC): amount of air that can be inhaled after normal expiration	Use direct spirographic measurement, or add IRV and VT.	Decreased IC indicates restrictive disease.

Interpreting pulmonary function tests *(continued)*

MEASUREMENT OF PULMONARY FUNCTION	METHOD OF CALCULATION	IMPLICATIONS
Thoracic gas volume (TGV): total volume of gas in lungs from both ventilated and nonventilated airways	Measure using body plethysmography.	Increased TGV indicates air trapping, which may result from obstructive disease.
Functional residual capacity (FRC): amount of air remaining in lungs after normal expiration	Measure using body plethysmography or helium dilution technique; or add ERV and RV.	Increased FRC indicates overdistended lungs, which may result from obstructive pulmonary disease.
Total lung capacity (TLC): total volume of the lungs when maximally inflated	Add VT, IRV, ERV, and RV; or add FRC and IC; or add VC and RV.	Low TLC indicates restrictive disease; high TLC indicates overdistended lungs caused by obstructive disease.
Forced vital capacity (FVC): the amount of air exhaled forcefully and quickly after maximum inspiration	Use direct spirographic measurement; expressed as a percentage of the total volume of gas exhaled.	Decreased FVC indicates flow resistance in respiratory system from obstructive disease, such as chronic bronchitis, or from restrictive disease, such as pulmonary fibrosis.
Flow-volume curve [also called flow-volume loop]: greatest rate of flow (Vmax) during FVC maneuvers versus lung volume change	Use direct spirographic measurement at 1-second intervals; calculated from flow rates (expressed in liters/second) and lung volume changes (expressed in liters) during maximal inspiratory and expiratory maneuvers.	Decreased flow rates at all volumes during expiration indicate obstructive disease of the small airways, such as emphysema. A plateau of expiratory flow near TLC, a plateau of inspiratory flow at mid-VC, and a square wave pattern through most of VC indicate obstructive disease of large airways. Normal or increased peak expiratory flow, decreased flow with decreasing lung volumes, and markedly decreased VC indicate restrictive disease.
Forced expiratory volume (FEV): volume of air expired in the first, second, or third second of FVC maneuver	Use direct spirographic measurement; expressed as percentage of FVC.	Decreased FEV_1, and increased FEV_2 and FEV_3 may indicate obstructive disease; decreased or normal FEV_1 may indicate restrictive disease.
Forced expiratory flow ($FEF_{25\%-75\%}$): average rate of flow during middle half of FVC	Calculate from the flow rate and the time needed for expiration of middle 50% of FVC.	Low $FEF_{25\%-75\%}$ indicates obstructive disease of the small airways.

(continued)

Interpreting pulmonary function tests *(continued)*

MEASUREMENT OF PULMONARY FUNCTION	METHOD OF CALCULATION	IMPLICATIONS
Peak expiratory flow (PEF): Vmax during forced expiration	Calculate from flow-volume curve, or by direct spirographic measurement, using a pneumotachometer or electronic tachometer with a transducer to convert flow to electrical output display.	Decreased PEF may indicate a mechanical problem, such as upper airway obstruction, or obstructive disease. PEF is usually normal in restrictive disease but decreases in severe cases. Because PEF is effort-dependent, it's also low in a person who has poor expiratory effort or doesn't understand the procedure.
Maximal voluntary ventilation (MVV) [also called maximum breathing capacity (MBC)]: greatest volume of air breathed per unit of time	Use direct spirographic measurement.	Decreased MVV may indicate obstructive disease; normal or decreased MVV may indicate restrictive disease, such as myasthenia gravis.

Attach the mask or mouthpiece to the spirometer, and instruct your patient to breathe normally. Insert the mouthpiece adapter into his mouth or place the mask over his mouth and nose. If your patient isn't intubated, use a nose clip to prevent air from entering through his nose, which would lower the tidal volume. If your patient has a tracheostomy or endotracheal tube, attach the spirometer to the tube. (See *Bedside tools for PFTs,* page 60).

Count 10 normal breaths, and note the clockwise movement of the spirometer needles. At the end of 10 breaths, turn off the spirometer and remove it from the patient. Divide the total volume you obtain by 10. This gives you the average tidal volume.

If you're assessing the patient's ability to be weaned, remove the ventilator. Then allow 30 to 60 seconds for his normal respiratory pattern to be established before attaching the spirometer to the tube. Be sure to monitor for pulse changes that may result from hypoxemia during the test. Resume mechanical ventilation at the end of the procedure or at any sign of respiratory distress.

Certain ventilators can continuously measure both inspiratory and expiratory tidal volume. To obtain a measurement, turn the selection knob to either inspiratory tidal volume or expiratory tidal volume. The value will appear on the digital display in milliliters.

Evaluating the results. Normal tidal volume is 5 to 7 ml/kg of ideal body weight. Expect to see a lower volume in a patient with restrictive lung disease, ventilatory muscle fatigue, or central nervous system (CNS) depression. Expect to see a higher volume with such disorders as metabolic acidosis, hypoxemia, and CNS stimulation.

Reading a spirogram

The plotting of a spirogram, or lung signature, is based on the following: the patient's tidal volume (VT) and his maximum inspiration (A) and expiration (B) capabilities, which constitute forced vital capacity (FVC). After these are plotted, a spirogram can be used to calculate inspiratory reserve volume (IRV), expiratory reserve volume (ERV), residual volume (RV), inspiratory capacity (IC), functional residual capacity (FRC), and total lung capacity (TLC).

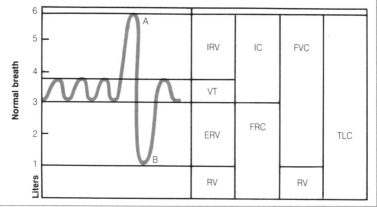

When using low-flow oxygen systems to determine the FIO_2, be sure to measure tidal volume. Remember, increases in tidal volume decrease the FIO_2 because of greater entrainment, resulting in more dilution with room air; decreases in tidal volume increase the FIO_2.

Minute volume

Minute volume is calculated by multiplying the tidal volume (in ml/breath) by the respiratory rate (breaths/minute). Certain ventilators can measure expiratory minute volume continuously. To obtain the measurement, turn the selection knob to expiratory minute volume; the value will appear on the digital display in liters per minute.

Evaluating the results. Normal minute volume for an adult is 5 to 10 liters. High minute volume indicates

an increase in demand. This results from excessive CO_2 production, which may occur with sepsis and fever and with disorders causing high dead-space ventilation — ARDS, COPD, and pulmonary embolism, for example.

You'll also use minute volume to determine whether a patient on mechanical ventilation can be weaned. If he can maintain a $PaCO_2$ of 40 mm Hg with a minute volume of less than 10 liters, he can probably be weaned successfully.

Vital capacity

For this test, prepare the Wright spirometer and your patient in the same way as for a tidal volume measurement. Remember, accurate results depend on patient cooperation.

Instruct the patient to take the deepest breath possible. Press the

Bedside tools for PFTs

The illustrations below show two common tools you'll use to perform bedside tests—the Wright spirometer and the inspiratory pressure manometer. Both are being used on a patient with a tracheostomy tube.

Wright spirometer

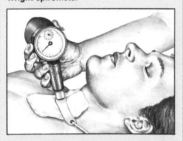

Inspiratory pressure manometer

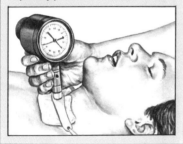

button on the spirometer quickly to reset the dial to zero. Then tell him to exhale until he feels that he has completely emptied his lungs. At the end of the exhalation, turn the control switch off so the measurement stays on the dial. This reading is the patient's vital capacity. After recording it, repeat the procedure at least twice to make sure you have an accurate measurement.

Evaluating the results. Normal vital

capacity is based on predicted values obtained from nomograms (see *Using nomograms for spirometry*). Expect to see decreased vital capacity in patients with restrictive lung disease who have a decreased total lung capacity. You'll also see decreased vital capacity in patients with obstructive lung disease who have an increased residual volume. Vital capacity will be reduced in patients on prolonged bed rest and in those with neuromuscular or musculoskeletal disorders, restrictive parenchymal diseases, recent chest or abdominal surgery, hypokalemia, or hypochloremia. A patient with a vital capacity below 10 ml/kg of body weight may need mechanical ventilation because of trouble clearing secretions, sighing, and taking deep breaths. Decreased vital capacity also appears in debilitated or malnourished patients.

Like minute volume, vital capacity should be used to determine if a patient can be weaned from a mechanical ventilator. If your patient has a vital capacity of 10 or more ml/kg of body weight, weaning should be successful.

Maximum inspiratory pressure
You'll use an inspiratory pressure manometer attached to the patient's airway to measure maximum inspiratory pressure. The device and an adapter can either be placed in your patient's mouth or connected to an endotracheal or tracheostomy tube. If your patient is intubated, make sure the manometer cuff is inflated.

Explain the procedure to your patient, and tell him he'll feel like he can't catch his breath during the 10 to 20 seconds you're actually measuring. Then tell him to breathe spontaneously for a few breaths. At the end of a normal exhalation,

Using nomograms for spirometry

Nomogram for men

With this nomogram for men, you can evaluate forced expiratory volume in ½ second ($FEV_{0.5}$), forced maximal voluntary ventilation (MVV_F), forced expiratory volume in 1 second ($FEV_{1.0}$), and vital capacity (VC). Just place a ruler so it intersects your patient's height and age. The points where the ruler intersects the other columns indicate the normal values for your patient. For instance, the line drawn here shows that a man who's 71″ tall and 30 years old should have a VC of 5.08 liters.

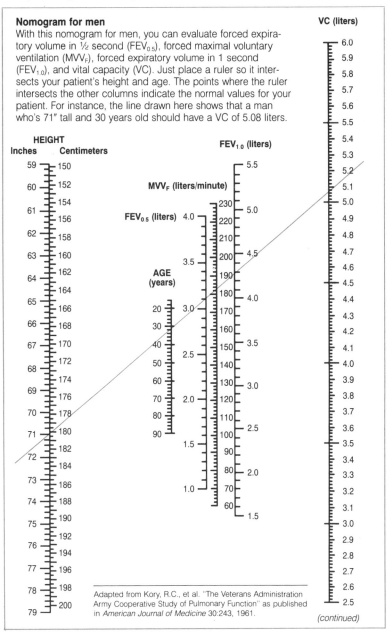

Adapted from Kory, R.C., et al. "The Veterans Administration Army Cooperative Study of Pulmonary Function" as published in *American Journal of Medicine* 30:243, 1961.

(continued)

Using nomograms for spirometry *(continued)*

Nomogram for women

With this nomogram for women, you can evaluate forced expiratory volume in ½ second ($FEV_{0.5}$), forced expiratory volume in 1 second ($FEV_{1.0}$), and forced vital capacity (FVC). The line drawn on the nomogram shows that a woman who's 64″ tall and 40 years old should have a $FEV_{1.0}$ of 2.9 liters, a $FEV_{0.5}$ of 2.2 liters, and a FVC of 3.3 liters.

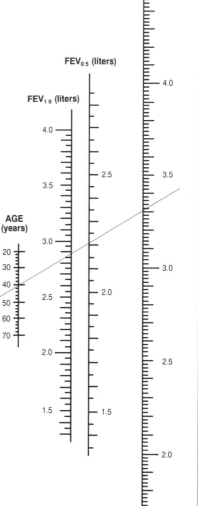

cover the manifold safety port with your thumb or fingertip to occlude the airway. Now tell the patient to inhale as deeply and with as much effort as possible. Keep the safety port occluded for 10 to 20 seconds, enough time for the patient to attempt inspiration. The red needle on the meter dial records the maximum inspiratory pressure with each inspiratory attempt. The black needle captures this reading, rising higher and locking with each greater exertion, so the best effort is recorded. After the patient has had a chance to rest and breathe normally, repeat the procedure to check the accuracy of the measurement.

Evaluating the results. A normal healthy adult should be able to generate a pressure of at least -80 cm H_2O. A pressure of less than -25 cm H_2O tells you that the patient needs mechanical ventilation. If the patient is already on mechanical ventilation and has a maximum inspiratory pressure of less than -20 cm H_2O, he probably can't be weaned successfully.

Inspiratory capacity

Prepare the Wright spirometer and the patient as you did for measuring tidal volume. Insert the spirometer into the patient's mouth or attach it to the tracheostomy or endotracheal tube. Instruct him to inhale to the end of a normal inspiration. Then press the reset button to return the hands on the dial to zero. Now tell your patient to continue to inhale until he feels he can't take in any more air. Turn the control switch off to record the measurement. Repeat the procedure to make sure your measurement is accurate.

Evaluating the results. Inspiratory capacity helps in choosing the appropriate type of delivery device for inhaled medications and in determining if incentive spirometry will be useful. To evaluate your patient's inspiratory capacity, you have to refer to a nomogram. If he needs inhaled medication and his inspiratory capacity is 40% or more, he can use a hand-held nebulizer. If his capacity is less than 40%, IPPB delivery will be more effective.

Incentive spirometry may help prevent pulmonary complications in a patient at risk. But this technique should be used only if the patient's inspiratory capacity is 40% or more.

Expiratory flow rates

Actually three measurements— forced vital capacity, forced expiratory volume, and forced expiratory flow—expiratory flow rates are based on one procedure.
• *Forced vital capacity.* The procedure for measuring forced vital capacity with a Wright spirometer is the same as for vital capacity except that you must instruct your patient to exhale as quickly, forcefully, and completely as possible. Repeat the procedure three times to make sure your measurement is accurate, letting your patient rest briefly between measurements.

If you're using a spirometer that provides a graphic recording, have your patient seal his lips around the mouthpiece, or attach the device to the endotracheal or tracheostomy tube. After he has breathed normally for about 1 minute, tell him to take as deep a breath as possible, to hold it for a short period, then to exhale as quickly, forcefully, and completely as possible. The pattern of exhalation will be recorded on the graph paper. Again, repeat this procedure three times.
• *Forced expiratory volume.* Testing for forced vital capacity also allows

you to measure the patient's forced expiratory volume. This is the amount of the forced vital capacity exhaled in 1, 2, or 3 seconds (FEV_1, FEV_2, FEV_3). You obtain these measurements from the graphic recording.

• *Forced expiratory flow.* Another measurement based on forced vital capacity is forced expiratory flow. It's determined from the flow rate and the time needed for expiration of the middle 50% of the forced vital capacity. You can get this measurement from the graphic recording.

Evaluating the results. To evaluate your patient's expiratory flow rates, again refer to a nomogram. Values below 80% are abnormal. Bedside monitoring of expiratory flow rates can help determine the efficacy of treatment. In a patient who has obstructive disease, the flow rates should improve with treatment. So you may take measurements both before and after your patient uses an aerosol bronchodilator to determine how well he's responding. If you find an improvement of 15% or more in the values—particularly in the FEV_2—you can consider his disease reversible. If the values don't improve, he has an irreversible disease; continuing bronchodilator therapy is contraindicated.

You can also use bedside monitoring to find out how long a drug is effective. To do so, measure expiratory flow rates every 30 to 60 minutes.

Peak expiratory flow

As a substitute for the graphic recording of forced expiratory volume and flow, you can measure peak expiratory flow, using a device such as the Wright peak-flow meter. To set the dial on the flow meter to

zero, press the release button. Then have the patient place his lips tightly around the mouthpiece, or attach the device to the endotracheal or tracheostomy tube. Instruct the patient to perform a forced vital capacity maneuver. The peak-flow meter will record a reading in liters per second or minute. Repeat this procedure twice to make sure your measurement is accurate.

Peak airway and plateau pressures

Although these measurements of airway resistance and lung compliance aren't always considered PFTs, they can indicate lung function. With a mechanically ventilated patient, you'll use these measurements to help determine ventilator adjustments and to monitor his condition. Because of the wide range of values obtained for patients who are being mechanically ventilated, noting baseline measurements isn't as useful as monitoring changes from the baseline.

Peak airway pressure depends on both the elastic properties of the respiratory system and the amount of resistance to airflow in the conducting airways. Plateau pressure, which is measured in the absence of airflow, is affected by the elastic properties but not by airflow obstruction.

Some ventilators measure peak airway and plateau pressures continuously. To obtain a reading, turn the selection knob to either peak airway pressure or plateau pressure and read the value on the digital display. If you have a ventilator that doesn't measure these pressures, use the water pressure manometer on the ventilator. You can obtain a plateau pressure by one of these three methods:

• Crimp the exhalation valve tubing

at end-inspiration and observe the fall in pressure to plateau. Once the plateau is reached, release the tubing.
• Occlude the expiratory port at the manifold at end-inspiration and observe the plateau pressure.
• Institute an inspiratory pause, observe the plateau pressure, and then discontinue the inspiratory pause.

No matter which of the three methods you use, make sure you complete the procedure within 3 seconds and monitor your patient for signs of barotrauma both during and immediately after the procedure.

The effective *dynamic compliance* is determined by the interaction of secretions or obstructions in the airways, the flow of gas into the airways, and the distensibility of the lungs. Dynamic compliance is calculated by subtracting PEEP from the peak airway pressure and dividing that into exhaled tidal volume. *Static compliance* is calculated by subtracting PEEP from the plateau pressure and then dividing that into exhaled tidal volume.

Evaluating the results. A decrease in static compliance suggests pneumothorax, atelectasis, pneumonia, pulmonary edema, or displacement of the endotracheal tube. A decrease in dynamic compliance may result from bronchospasm or retained secretions.

Static compliance measurements can help establish the best level of PEEP to administer to a patient with acute respiratory failure. Decreased static compliance indicates that a shunt is developing, and the patient will need PEEP to achieve adequate oxygenation; if it's effective, PEEP should increase static compliance. An increase in dynamic

or static compliance or both suggests an improvement in the underlying respiratory problem.

Additional tests

As part of assessing your patient's status, you may also have to calculate an intrapulmonary shunt or assist with a chest X-ray.

Calculating an intrapulmonary shunt

You can determine the degree of oxygen diffusion across the alveolo-capillary membrane through a series of calculations (see *How to calculate an intrapulmonary shunt,* pages 66 and 67). In most cases, a calculated shunt exceeding 30% is considered incompatible with prolonged spontaneous ventilation. The patient would require mechanical ventilation to maintain adequate tissue oxygenation. For a patient already on mechanical ventilation, weaning would probably be unsuccessful if the shunt exceeded 15%.

Chest X-rays

Chest X-rays are routinely taken to assess pulmonary status. Serial films can help monitor patients with such disorders as pneumonia, ARDS, pneumothorax, hemothorax, and atelectasis. Such film can also help monitor a patient's response to treatment. You'll see chest X-rays ordered to check the placement of central lines and endotracheal tubes.

Before a bedside chest X-ray using a portable machine, help place the patient in high Fowler's position. This position will facilitate optimal lung expansion and descent of the diaphragm. If your patient

How to calculate an intrapulmonary shunt

By using one of the following methods, you can determine your patient's intrapulmonary shunt at bedside.

Calculating a shunt from venous blood samples

The most accurate method requires samples of blood drawn simultaneously for measurement of arterial blood gas levels, hemoglobin (Hb) concentration, and mixed venous oxygen and carbon dioxide levels. (The mixed venous blood sample must be drawn from the distal lumen of the pulmonary artery catheter.)

To obtain data for the equations, administer high concentrations of oxygen for 15 to 30 minutes before collecting the blood samples. Usually, 50% oxygen is adequate; however, some doctors may specify 100% oxygen, the previously recommended level.

You can then calculate the shunt and the oxygen content of perfused and ventilated pulmonary capillary blood (CcO_2) by applying the collected data to the following equations:

$$CcO_2 = (Hb \times 1.34) + (PaO_2 \times 0.003)$$

$$CaO_2 = \frac{(Hb \times 1.34 \times \% \text{ saturation})}{100} + (PaO_2 \times 0.003)$$

$$CvO_2 = \frac{(Hb \times 1.34 \times \% \text{ saturation}}{100} + (PvO_2) \times 0.003)$$

Shunted blood, expressed as a ratio of the total blood flow (Qs/Qt), can then be calculated as shown here:

$$\frac{Qs}{Qt} = \frac{(CcO_2 - CaO_2)}{(CcO_2 - CvO_2)}$$

can't sit upright, place him in the supine position. With this position, however, fluid levels in the pleural space won't be visualized.

Most commonly, the posteroanterior view will be used for bedside X-rays. The film is placed behind the patient's back and the X-ray beam directed toward him. Once the film is in place, make sure that all cardiac monitoring cables, ventilator tubing, I.V. tubing from central lines, safety pins, ECG leads, and jewelry are moved as far out of the way as possible. If your patient is pregnant or suspects she may be, place a lead apron over her abdomen. To avoid extra exposure to radiation yourself, leave the room while the X-ray is being taken. If you must stay in the area, wear a lead apron.

The chest X-rays will show what anatomic changes the disease process or medical intervention has caused, and that can help you plan your interventions.

Suggested readings

Briones, T.L. "SvO$_2$ Monitoring: Part I, Clinical Case Application," *DCCN* 7(2):70-78, April 1988.

Carlon, G.C., et al. "Capnography in

Calculating a shunt from oxygen content

A simpler calculation uses partial pressures for oxygen content. It assumes that hemoglobin is fully saturated with oxygen.

$$\frac{Qs}{Qt} = \frac{([PAO_2 - PaO_2]\ 0.003)}{(CaO_2 - CvO_2) + (PAO_2 - PaO_2)\ 0.003}$$

Calculating a shunt from alveolar-arterial (A-a) gradient

This method is less accurate than the others because it doesn't account for cardiac output changes. However, it's faster and easier to use for bedside monitoring. The equation compares estimated partial pressure of oxygen in alveolar blood (PAO_2) with partial pressure of oxygen in arterial blood (PaO_2). The result (difference) is known as the A-a gradient:

$$A\text{-a gradient} = PAO_2 - PaO_2$$

Then, to estimate the degree of shunting when the patient is breathing 100% oxygen, use this equation:

$$\%\ \text{shunt} = \frac{(P[A\text{-a}]O_2)}{100} \times 5\%$$

Calculating a shunt from arterial-alveolar (a-A) ratio

You may prefer to assess your patient's shunt by calculating the a-A ratio because this value varies with the $PaCO_2$ level and the ventilation-perfusion ratio but not with FIO_2. Use this equation:

$$a\text{-A ratio} = \frac{PaO_2}{PAO_2}$$

Mechanically Ventilated Patients,'' *Critical Care Medicine* 16(5):550-56, May 1988.

Kinney, M.R., et al. *AACN'S Clinical Reference for Critical-Care Nursing*, 2nd ed. New York: McGraw-Hill Book Co., 1987.

Sanders, A.B. ''Capnometry in Emergency Medicine,'' *Annals of Emergency Medicine* 18(12):1287-90, December 1989.

Schroeder, C.H. ''Pulse Oximetry: A Nursing Care Plan,'' *Critical Care Nurse* 8(8):50-66, November-December 1988.

Spyr, J., and Preach, M.A. ''Pulse Oximetry: Understanding the Concept, Knowing the Limits,'' *RN* 53(5):38-45, May 1990.

Stewart, F.M. ''SvO_2 Monitoring: Part II, Nursing Research Applications,'' *DCCN* 7(2):79-82, April 1988.

3

AIRWAY MAINTENANCE

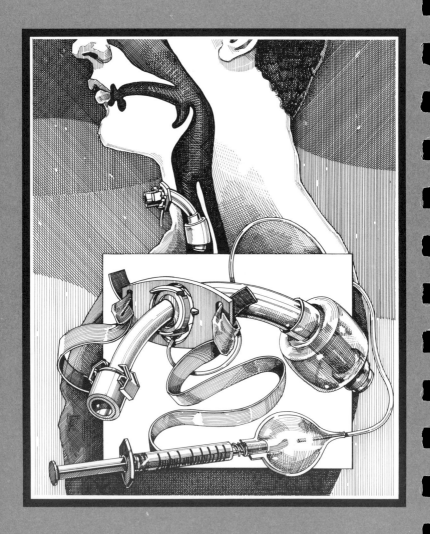

Like most aspects of respiratory care, the methods used to establish and maintain a patent airway have changed over the past decade. These new methods — along with advances in home therapy, equipment, and treatment techniques — have greatly improved the quality of care respiratory patients receive.

This chapter acquaints you with certain equipment innovations — such as more flexible plastic tubes, high-volume/low-pressure cuffs, and disposable equipment. The chapter also discusses advances in maintaining adequate humidification and tracheostomy care. And you'll read about certain improved techniques for performing procedures, such as inflating an endotracheal tube cuff using the minimal leak or minimal occlusive volume technique, and suctioning with less trauma to the patient's trachea and upper airway.

But the focus of this chapter is procedures — some basic, such as chest physiotherapy; others more difficult, such as artificial airway insertion. As you read about them, keep in mind that despite all the innovations, one thing about airway maintenance remains the same. The success of the procedures depends largely on your skills and expertise.

Chest physiotherapy

Increased respiratory secretions commonly result in airway obstruction — especially in patients with pneumonia, cystic fibrosis, bronchiectasis, or chronic obstructive pulmonary disease (COPD); those who may be immobilized, weak, or debilitated; and those with a neuro-muscular disease that prevents effective movement of secretions. You can help prevent obstructions in these patients using the various components of chest physiotherapy discussed here.

A collective term, chest physiotherapy encompasses five treatments to clear the patient's airways: coughing, deep breathing, positioning and postural drainage, percussion, and vibration. Chest physiotherapy mobilizes and eliminates secretions from the airways, helps prevent alveolar collapse or reexpands alveoli, and promotes efficient use of respiratory muscles. Especially in bedridden patients, these treatments play a vital role in helping prevent or treat atelectasis and pneumonia — respiratory complications that can seriously impede recovery.

Indications and contraindications

Chest physiotherapy may be used when a patient has secretions associated with bronchitis, cystic fibrosis, bronchiectasis, or pneumonia; a disease that causes neuromuscular weakness (Guillain-Barré syndrome, myasthenia gravis, tetanus); COPD (emphysema); a disease associated with aspiration (cerebral palsy or muscular dystrophy); or postoperative pain associated with impaired breathing (thoracic or abdominal incisions). You may also use it on a patient with prolonged immobility.

Chest physiotherapy is contraindicated during active pulmonary bleeding with hemoptysis as well as during the post-hemorrhage stage. Other contraindications include fractured ribs, an unstable chest wall, lung contusions, pulmonary tuberculosis, untreated pneumothorax, acute asthma or bronchospasm, lung abscess or tumor, head injury, and recent myocardial infarction.

Basic care

Before chest physiotherapy, be sure to tell the patient what to expect and what's expected of him. Auscultate his lungs to obtain baseline findings. For a postoperative patient, give an analgesic, as ordered, and wait for it to take effect before beginning coughing and deep breathing.

During treatment, assess the patient's tolerance of the procedures and monitor him for adverse reactions. Have him cough afterward to remove loosened secretions. Also, auscultate his lungs again to determine the effectiveness of treatment.

Expect to modify chest physiotherapy according to your patient's condition. For example, you'll administer supplemental oxygen to a hypoxic patient or suction a patient with an ineffective cough reflex. If the patient weakens rapidly during chest physiotherapy, switch to shorter, more frequent sessions. Keep in mind that fatigue leads to shallow respirations and worsened hypoxia.

Any adjunct therapy — such as intermittent positive-pressure breathing (IPPB), aerosol, or nebulizer treatment — should precede chest physiotherapy. Make sure your patient stays adequately hydrated, which will help dilute secretions and ease mobilization.

Coughing

Performed with deep-breathing exercises, coughing helps prevent obstruction by keeping the patient's airways clear and open. Coughing dislodges and removes secretions from the pulmonary tree, while deep breathing increases air in the alveoli, making the cough more effective.

Your patient may think he already knows how to cough, but the techniques you teach him will make him cough more effectively. An effective cough sounds deep, low, and hollow; an ineffective cough sounds high-pitched.

To teach the patient to cough effectively, follow these steps:
• Make sure he's in a comfortable, upright position, then have him inhale deeply through his nose and exhale in three short huffs.
• Now have him inhale deeply and cough three times with his mouth slightly open.
• Repeat the exercise two or three times.

When a patient can't cough effectively, try teaching him one of the following techniques.

Cascade cough. When the patient has the strength to cough, no bronchospasm, and airways that don't collapse, the cascade cough may help make his coughing more effective.

Have him take three to four deep breaths, exhaling slowly through his mouth. During exhalation of the last breath, have him perform a staged series of three to four coughs.

Huff cough. Teach the patient to use the huff cough when bronchospasm is present, when the airways might collapse, or when the patient seems afraid to perform the cascade cough, perhaps because of postoperative pain. Here's how to proceed:
• Have him take two to three slow, deep breaths.
• Then have him take one to two slow, deep breaths, exhaling in three short bursts or huffs.
• Finally, have him take a deep breath and exhale in faster, more forceful bursts with the glottis open, producing three to four strong huffs until exhalation is complete.

Cough-friendly technique. Have the patient use the cough-friendly technique when he doesn't have the strength in his chest wall, diaphragm, or abdomen to produce a forceful cough. To use this technique, follow these steps:

• With the patient seated and his feet on the floor or a stool, place a pillow or blanket over his abdomen that he can support with his forearms. Tell him to bend forward, pressing his forearms against his abdomen and exhaling. Have him return to the sitting position, inhaling deeply through his nose. Repeat the cycle two to three times.

• After the last breath, have the patient cough two to three times while bending forward and pressing firmly on his abdomen.

Quad cough. When the patient can take a deep breath but can't generate enough force for a cough, have him use the quad cough. Follow these steps:

• With the patient supine and the head of the bed elevated 45 degrees or less, have him take two to three slow, deep breaths, exhaling slowly through his mouth.

• While he takes a deep breath, place the palm of your hand on his abdomen above the umbilicus and below the ribs. As he exhales and tries to cough, press sharply inward and upward two to three times.

Nursing considerations. Teach a surgical or trauma patient with chest wall or abdominal pain to splint his incision or painful area when he coughs. Have him place one hand above the area and one hand below it, or hold a pillow or towel roll against the area. You can also splint the site when he coughs.

Auscultate the patient's lungs before and after coughing to evaluate the effectiveness of therapy.

Regardless of the coughing technique used, have the patient take three slow, deep breaths and allow him to rest briefly between repetitions. Tell him never to suppress a spontaneous cough that occurs during treatment. Be sure to provide oral hygiene after coughing therapy because secretions may taste foul or have a stale odor.

Deep breathing

After coughing, the patient should breathe deeply to increase the amount of air in his lungs to help prevent alveolar collapse or reexpand collapsed alveoli. Exhaling through pursed lips temporarily encourages a slow, deep breathing pattern; reduces partial pressure of carbon dioxide in arterial blood ($PaCO_2$) and improves partial pressure of oxygen in arterial blood (PaO_2); and decreases the work of breathing. Abdominal contraction pushes the diaphragm upward, exerts pressure on the lungs, and helps empty the alveoli. If the patient has COPD, causing chronic retention of carbon dioxide, diaphragmatic breathing and pursed-lip breathing may be especially helpful.

To teach your patient to breathe deeply, follow these steps:

• With the patient seated or supine and the head of his bed elevated, have him put one hand on the middle of his chest and the other on his abdomen, just below his ribs, to feel his diaphragm rise and fall.

• Instruct the patient to inhale slowly and deeply, pushing his abdomen out against his hand to provide optimal distribution of air to the alveoli. Tell him to exhale through pursed lips, contracting his abdomen at the same time.

• Have the patient breathe this way for 1 minute and then rest for 2

IPPB: The pros and cons

Although most hospitals use incentive spirometry to prevent pulmonary complications, some use intermittent positive-pressure breathing (IPPB) treatments, which deliver a mixture of air and oxygen to the lungs at a preset pressure. IPPB works by:
• expanding airways
• loosening secretions
• delivering aerosol medications.

Ineffective or improper treatment
Despite these benefits, IPPB isn't always effective. For example, a patient who finds treatments frightening or painful (because of lung expansion) may decrease air delivery to the lungs by putting his tongue in front of the mouthpiece. This lets the air fill his cheeks instead of his lungs and diminishes the volume of the air available to inflate alveoli. And, although IPPB easily inflates healthy alveoli, it may have little effect on alveoli with thickened or obstructed walls—the walls most difficult to inflate. If a patient receives IPPB without close supervision, hyperventilation may occur, resulting in respiratory alkalosis and dizziness. If administered inappropriately, IPPB can cause cardiac output to drop suddenly, leading to tachycardia, dyspnea, and anxiety.

Risks of treatment
IPPB can also pose health risks. For example, swallowing air during the treatments may produce gastric insufflation, putting the patient at greater risk of developing stress ulcers, especially if he's NPO over 24 hours.

fully cooperating with breathing exercises, incentive spirometry can help prevent pulmonary complications, such as atelectasis or pneumonia. Incentive spirometry increases a patient's lung expansion while objectively evaluating his deep breathing. Many clinicians consider it safer and more effective than IPPB. (See *IPPB: The pros and cons.*)

Normally, people sigh every 6 to 10 minutes, but when the sighing produces pain, people naturally override the process and take only shallow breaths that do little to clear the airways. Incentive spirometry replaces this natural sighing, inducing the patient to take a deep breath and hold it. Then, the spirometer measures the amount of air inhaled.

Using the incentive spirometer, you and the patient can gauge his progress by setting goals to reach or to maintain. (Some incentive spirometers can be adjusted to increase the degree of difficulty so the patient always works toward improvement.)

To use the incentive spirometer, follow these steps:
• Help the patient to a sitting position to promote optimal lung expansion.
• Instruct him to exhale normally, then place his lips tightly around the mouthpiece of the incentive spirometer and inhale deeply. Unless ordered otherwise, encourage him to inhale deeply enough to force the ball to the chamber top, to compress the bellows, or to light up the different color panels, as indicated by the specific incentive spirometer you're using.

If the patient has difficulty achieving this goal, tell him to suck in as if he were sipping through a straw. Inspiring slowly ensures

minutes. Gradually progress to a 10-minute exercise period four times a day.

Incentive spirometry. When associated pain prevents a patient from an even distribution of air to the alveoli.

• Note the maximum volume of air the patient inhales, called the inspiratory capacity. (Some machines will automatically record the highest level reached.)

• After inspiration, have the patient hold his breath for 3 seconds, then remove the mouthpiece and exhale normally.

• The patient should repeat the exercise 5 to 10 times per hour. A 60-second rest between consecutive deep breaths will help prevent fatigue and dizziness.

Nursing considerations. Assure your patient that holding one deep breath for a few seconds will be more effective in preventing pulmonary complications than taking several deep breaths and immediately exhaling.

When planning coughing and deep-breathing exercises, keep in mind that any pain will reduce the patient's effort.

Postural drainage

Follow coughing and deep-breathing exercises with postural drainage to help clear obstructed airways. Performed in conjunction with percussion and vibration treatments, postural drainage is the sequential positioning of the patient so that gravity can drain the peripheral pulmonary secretions into the major bronchi or trachea. Secretions usually drain best from bronchi positioned perpendicular to the floor. Lower and middle lobe bronchi usually empty best in the head-down position; upper lobe bronchi, in the head-up position. Chest X-ray results and auscultation findings determine the best position for the patient to assume.

In generalized disease, drainage usually begins with the lower lobes, continues with the middle lobes, and ends with the upper lobes. In localized disease, drainage begins with the affected lobes and then proceeds with the other lobes to avoid spreading the disease to uninvolved areas.

To perform postural drainage, follow these steps:

• Place the patient in the position that most effectively loosens and drains the affected area (see *Positioning patients for postural drainage,* pages 74 and 75).

• Have the patient remain in each position for 10 to 15 minutes while you perform percussion and vibration, as ordered.

Nursing considerations. To avoid nausea and aspiration of food or vomitus, wait 1½ hours after the patient eats before performing postural drainage.

Percussion

Performed by percussing the chest with cupped hands, this procedure mechanically dislodges thick, tenacious secretions from the bronchial walls so they can be expectorated or suctioned.

To perform percussion, follow these steps:

• Instruct the patient to breathe slowly and deeply, using the diaphragm to promote relaxation.

• Cup your hands and percuss each lung segment for 1 to 2 minutes, rhythmically alternating your hands (see *Hand positions for percussion and vibration,* page 76). Listen for a hollow sound to gauge the effectiveness of your technique.

Nursing considerations. Percuss over bare skin. That way, the air cushion your hands create on contact will

(Text continues on page 76.)

Positioning patients for postural drainage

The following illustrations show you the various postural drainage positions and the areas of the lungs affected by each.

Lower lobes: Posterior basal segments

Elevate the foot of the bed 30 degrees. With the patient on his abdomen and his head lowered, position pillows under his chest and abdomen. Percuss his lower ribs on both sides of his spine.

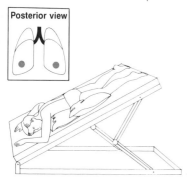

Posterior view

Lower lobes: Lateral basal segments

Elevate the foot of the bed 30 degrees. Instruct the patient to lie on his abdomen with his head lowered and his upper leg flexed over a pillow for support. Then have him rotate a quarter turn upward. Percuss his lower ribs on the uppermost portion of his lateral chest wall.

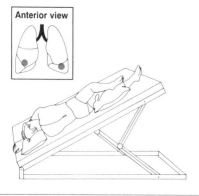

Anterior view

Lower lobes: Anterior basal segments

Elevate the foot of the bed 30 degrees. Instruct the patient to lie on his side with his head lowered. Then place pillows as shown below. Percuss with a slightly cupped hand over his lower ribs just beneath the axilla. *Note:* If an acutely ill patient experiences breathing difficulty in this position, adjust the angle of the bed to one he can tolerate. Then begin percussion.

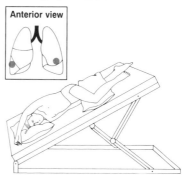

Anterior view

Lower lobes: Superior segments

With the bed flat, have the patient lie on his abdomen. Place two pillows under his hips. Percuss on both sides of his spine at the lower tip of his scapulae.

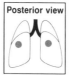

Posterior view

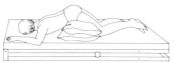

Right middle lobe: Medial and lateral segments

Elevate the foot of the bed 15 degrees, as shown at the top of the next column.

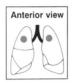

Anterior view

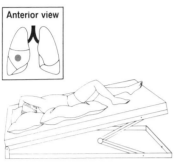

Have the patient lie on his left side with his head lowered and his knees flexed. Then have him rotate a quarter turn backward. Place a pillow beneath him. Percuss with your hand moderately cupped over the right nipple. In females, cup your hand so that its heel is under the armpit and your fingers extend forward beneath her breast.

Left upper lobe: Superior and inferior segments, lingular portion
Elevate the foot of the bed 15 degrees. Have the patient lie on his right side with his head lowered and knees flexed. Then have him rotate a quarter turn backward. Place a pillow behind him, from shoulders to hips. Percuss with your hand moderately cupped over his left nipple. In females, cup your hand so that its heel is beneath the armpit and your fingers extend forward beneath the breast.

Anterior view

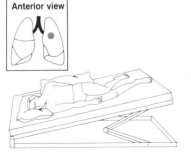

Upper lobes: Anterior segments
Make sure the bed is flat. Instruct the patient to lie on his back with a pillow folded under his knees, as shown below. Then have him rotate slightly away from the side being drained. Percuss between his clavicle and nipple.

Anterior view

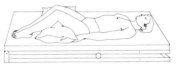

Upper lobes: Apical segments
Keep the bed flat. Have the patient lean back at a 30-degree angle against you and a pillow. Percuss with a cupped hand between his clavicles and the top of each scapula.

Posterior view

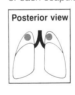
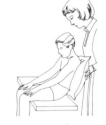

Upper lobes: Posterior segments
Keep the bed flat. Have the patient lean over a pillow at a 30-degree angle. Percuss and clap his upper back on each side.

Posterior view

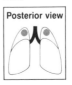

Hand positions for percussion and vibration

Percussion
To perform percussion, cup your hands with your fingers flexed and your thumb tight against your index finger.

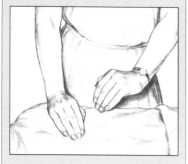

Vibration
To perform vibration, place your hands flat on the lung segment being drained. Position your hands side by side, with your fingers extended.

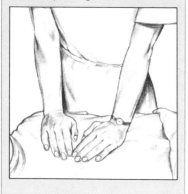

patient or a patient with poor skin turgor by percussing over the gown, other soft clothing, or a thin towel — not on bare skin. Don't percuss over buttons, snaps, or zippers, and remove any jewelry that may scratch or bruise the patient. To prevent injury, avoid percussing over the spine, liver, kidneys, spleen, or the female patient's breasts. To prevent rib fracture and pneumothorax, don't percuss too vigorously.

Vibration
Use vibration during postural drainage, either with percussion or as an alternative to it for a patient who's frail, in pain, or recovering from thoracic surgery or trauma. Vibration increases the velocity and turbulence of exhaled air, loosens secretions, and propels them into the larger bronchi so they can be expectorated or suctioned.

To perform vibration, follow these steps:
• Instruct the patient to inhale deeply and exhale slowly through pursed lips. During exhalation, firmly press your hands flat against his chest wall.
• Vibrate the patient's chest wall by quickly contracting and relaxing the muscles of your arms and shoulders to generate fine vibrations. Stop vibrating when he inhales. Vibrate during five exhalations over each lung segment.

send vibrations through the chest wall and help dislodge secretions from the bronchial wall. If redness or petechiae appear on the patient's skin, you may need to change your technique.

Prevent skin trauma in an elderly

Establishing an airway

Food lodged in the airway accounts for most obstructions among conscious patients. In unconscious or anesthetized patients, most obstructions occur when the tongue falls back and blocks the hypopharynx. Other causes of airway obstruction include laryngeal or bronchial spasm, infections, tumors, edema (from an allergy, burns, or extubation), trauma, foreign objects, and tracheal collapse.

A conscious patient with a complete upper airway obstruction will clutch his throat and be unable to speak. He'll fall unconscious within a few seconds. If an airway isn't established, you won't detect air exchange and irreversible brain damage will follow within 6 minutes.

Although less dramatic, the signs and symptoms of a partial or impending airway obstruction are equally unmistakable. Expect to see stridor on inspiration, exaggerated chest movements, muffled voice sounds, nasal flaring, tachycardia, restlessness, agitation, anxiety, and ashen, pallid, or cyanotic skin.

Emergency interventions, such as abdominal thrusts (Heimlich maneuver), finger sweep, and chest thrust, may remove the obstruction. (See *Managing an airway obstruction,* pages 78 to 81.) When emergency interventions fail, an artificial airway can be inserted in the nasopharynx or oropharynx, or an endotracheal or tracheostomy tube can be inserted to establish an airway and allow for deep suctioning and mechanical ventilation. If distal airways remain occluded, the doctor may perform bronchoscopy to remove a foreign body and establish a patent airway. In an emergency, if the obstruction can't be treated by opening the airway at a higher level, the patient may need either transtracheal catheter ventilation or an emergency cricothyrotomy.

Nasopharyngeal airway
Made of soft rubber or latex, a nasopharyngeal airway follows the curvature of the nasopharynx. This airway is passed through the patient's nose and extends from the nostril to the posterior pharynx. The bevel-shaped pharyngeal end eases insertion; the funnel-shaped nasal end helps prevent the airway from slipping. (See *Comparing artificial airways,* pages 82 and 83.)

Indications. A nasopharyngeal airway is indicated to prevent or relieve a soft-tissue upper airway obstruction when an oropharyngeal airway is contraindicated. A nasopharyngeal airway is also used to protect the nasal mucosa when a patient requires frequent suctioning and to maintain airway patency until a patient recovers from anesthesia. Contraindications include a predisposition to nosebleed, a nasal obstruction, a hemorrhagic disorder, and sepsis.

Insertion. Begin by gathering the following equipment: a nasopharyngeal airway, clean gloves, scissors, a ruler, a tongue depressor, and water-soluble lubricant. Then follow these steps:
• Wash your hands and put on the gloves. If time permits, explain the procedure to the patient.
• Measure the diameter of the patient's nostril and the distance from the tip of his nose to his earlobe. Select an airway that has a diameter slightly smaller than the nostril and cut it slightly longer than the length from the nose to the earlobe (about 1″ [2.5 cm] longer).
• Apply the water-soluble lubricant to the exterior of the airway to prevent trauma during insertion. If possible, use lidocaine gel because its anesthetic properties on the mucosa will make insertion more comfortable.

(Text continues on page 81.)

Managing an airway obstruction

Even when a patient shows the universal sign of an airway obstruction — clutching his throat with his mouth open — emergency intervention may not be necessary. Instead, intervention depends on several variables, including the patient's degree of consciousness and his ability to speak. To know how and when to intervene, follow these guidelines issued by the American Heart Association.

Clearing the airway
If a person shows signs of an obstruction, ask him if he can speak. If he answers — or if he coughs and chokes — his airway is partially open. In this case, don't interfere. Stand by and provide reassurance; he may be able to clear the airway himself.

If the patient can't speak, or if you note extreme breathing difficulty, stridor, a weak or ineffective cough, or cyanosis, intervene immediately. Standing behind the patient, support him with one arm. If possible, position his head below his shoulders to take advantage of gravitational force. Then cup your hand and deliver four sharp blows over his spine between the scapulae.

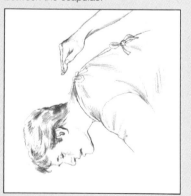

If these measures don't work, perform abdominal thrusts. Standing behind the patient, wrap both arms around his waist. Place your fist in the center of his abdomen, midway between the umbilicus and the xiphoid process. Rest the thumb side of your fist against his epigastrium and then grasp your fist with your other hand. Using a quick motion, thrust your fists inward and upward four times.

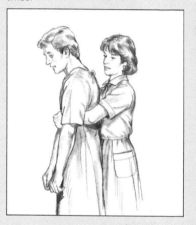

Alternate back blows with abdominal thrusts until you clear the airway or the patient loses consciousness. *Note:* Don't continue to give abdominal thrusts if a previous thrust has cleared the airway.

If the patient loses consciousness, ease him to the floor and call for help. If he's unconscious when you find him, first try rousing him. To do this and to protect yourself from injury, firmly grasp his upper arms, as shown at the top of the next column. This limits his range of motion if his arms begin to flail. Then, if you don't suspect a spinal cord injury, shake him and call his name.

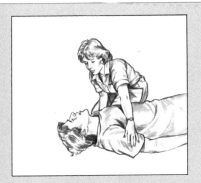

close to the back of his head. Gently press back on his forehead while lifting and supporting his neck.

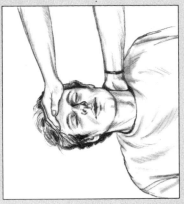

If the patient doesn't respond, call for help and position him flat on his back. If you don't suspect a spinal cord injury, open his airway with the head-tilt, chin-lift technique. To tilt the head, place one hand on his forehead, tilting it slightly back. Place the fingertips of your other hand under his lower jaw, on the bony part near his chin, and lift gently, taking care not to close his mouth.

If you suspect a spinal cord injury, use the jaw-thrust technique. Kneel at the patient's head, facing his feet. Place your thumbs on his jaw near the corners of his mouth, pointing your thumbs toward his feet. Then, position the tips of your index fingers at the angles of his jaw and push your thumbs down while you lift upward with the tips of your index fingers.

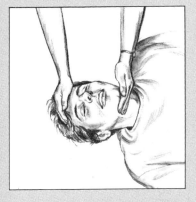

Alternatively, use the neck-lift technique. Place one hand on the patient's forehead and the other under his neck,

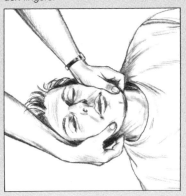

(continued)

Managing an airway obstruction *(continued)*

Assessing for breathing
Check for restored breathing by placing your ear slightly above the patient's mouth and nose. Listen for breath sounds, note any air movement against your cheek, and watch his chest and abdomen for movement.

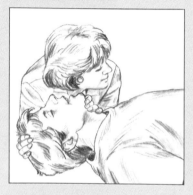

If the patient still isn't breathing, try to ventilate him by pinching his nose, placing your mouth over his, and blowing in air. If this isn't successful, reposition the patient's airway and try to ventilate again. If your second attempt doesn't succeed, assume he has a blocked airway.

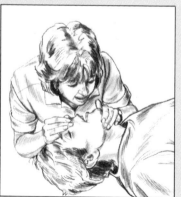

Logroll the patient toward you, and brace your thigh against his chest. With a cupped hand, deliver four sharp back blows between his scapulae.

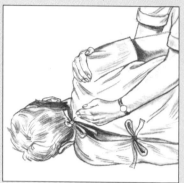

Roll the patient onto his back. Depending on your size and the patient's, kneel astride his hips or at his side.

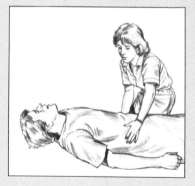

Place one hand on top of the other and lock your fingers. Then place the heel of your bottom hand over the epigastrium (above the umbilicus, but below the xiphoid process), as shown at the top of the next column. With four quick thrusts, press the heel of your bottom hand inward and upward, toward the patient's head.

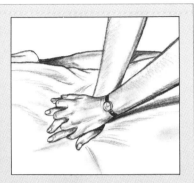

Open the patient's mouth and pull down his lower lip to look for an obstructing object or substance. If you see an obstruction, try to remove it, using the finger-sweep technique.

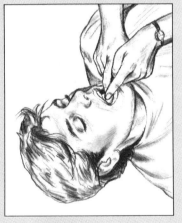

Now reposition his head and attempt to ventilate him. Continue to deliver abdominal thrusts and rescue breaths until breathing is restored or a tracheotomy becomes necessary.

• Hyperextend the patient's neck, if not contraindicated. Push up the tip of his nose and pass the airway into his nostril. Avoid pushing when you meet resistance to prevent tissue trauma and airway kinking.
• Check to see if the airway is positioned correctly by closing the patient's mouth and placing your finger in front of the opening to detect air exchange. Then use a tongue depressor to examine the airway tip behind the uvula.
• Properly dispose of the gloves and wash your hands.
• Auscultate the patient's lungs to ensure adequate ventilation.
• If the patient coughs or gags, the tube may be too long. If so, remove the airway and insert a shorter one.
• To increase oxygen availability during respiration, place a nasal cannula just under his nose. Rarely, a nasal cathetcr may be inserted.

Routine care. To prevent mucus from creating an obstruction, administer humidified oxygen and maintain adequate hydration. If the patient has secretions, try to get him to cough forcefully. If that doesn't remove the secretions, suction the patient's posterior pharynx to stimulate involuntary coughing.

Check the nasopharyngeal airway regularly to detect dislodgment or obstruction. To clean the airway, first remove it as described below. Place it in a basin and rinse it first with hydrogen peroxide and then with water. Use a pipe cleaner to remove any remaining secretions.

Inspect the skin around the nostrils for breakdown and the mucous membranes of the nose for trauma. If you detect breakdown or trauma, reinsert the clean airway into the other nostril if it's patent. Thoroughly document the procedure and your care measures.

Comparing artificial airways

Artificial airways come in five basic types: nasopharyngeal, oropharyngeal, nasal endotracheal, oral endotracheal, and tracheostomy. The following chart compares the advantages and disadvantages of each type.

AIRWAY	ADVANTAGES	DISADVANTAGES
Nasopharyngeal 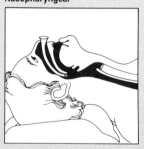	• Easily inserted • Better tolerated by conscious patients than oropharyngeal airway • Won't displace patient's nasal turbinates during suctioning	• May cause severe epistaxis if inserted too forcefully • May kink and clog, obstructing the airway • May cause pressure necrosis of nasal mucosa • May cause airway obstruction if artificial airway is too large
Oropharyngeal 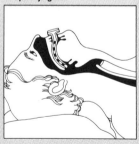	• Easily inserted • Holds tongue away from pharynx	• Easily dislodged • May stimulate gag reflex • May cause obstruction if wrong size airway is used • May not be tolerated well by conscious patients
Nasal endotracheal 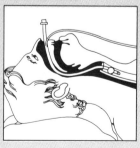	• More comfortable than oral endotracheal tube • Permits good oral hygiene • Can't be bitten or chewed • Provides a channel for suctioning • May be adapted easily if patient requires continuous ventilation • May be anchored in place easily • Prevents aspiration of stomach contents if cuff is inflated	• May lacerate pharyngeal mucosa or larynx during insertion • Kinks and clogs easily • Increases airway resistance because of small lumen size needed to fit nasal passages • May cause pressure necrosis, middle ear infection, laryngeal edema, or tracheal damage

EQUIPMENT

Comparing artificial airways *(continued)*

AIRWAY	ADVANTAGES	DISADVANTAGES
Oral endotracheal 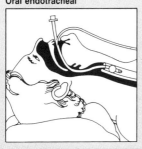	• Allows quick, easy insertion • Causes less intubation trauma than nasal endotracheal airway or tracheostomy tube • Prevents aspiration of stomach contents if cuff is inflated	• May damage teeth, lips, mouth, pharyngeal mucosa, or larynx during insertion • Activates gag reflex in conscious patients • Kinks and clogs easily • May be bitten or chewed • May cause pressure necrosis, middle ear infection, laryngeal edema, or tracheal damage
Tracheostomy 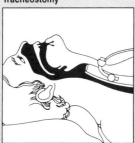	• Suctioned more easily than endotracheal tube • Reduces dead air space in respiratory tract • Causes less trauma to airways • Permits patient to swallow and eat more easily • More comfortable than other tubes • Prevents aspiration of stomach contents, if cuff is inflated	• Requires surgery to insert • May cause laceration or pressure necrosis of trachea • May cause tracheoesophageal fistula • Increases risk of tracheal and stomal inflammation, infection, and mucus plugs

Complications. A nasopharyngeal airway can cause nosebleed, pressure necrosis of the nasal mucosa, and sinus infection that results from sinus blockage.

If bleeding occurs, suction the airway until it's clear, then remove the airway as described below and clean it. Notify the doctor before reinserting the airway. If bleeding persists or recurs, or if skin breakdown and necrosis develop, discontinue using the airway.

Removing the airway. Before re-moving a nasopharyngeal airway, evaluate the patient's condition. Is his natural airway patent? If so, wash your hands, put on gloves, and pull out the nasopharyngeal airway in one smooth motion. If the airway sticks, apply lubricant around the nasal end of the tube and around the nostril; gently rotate the airway until you can pull it free.

After removing the tube, clean the area around the nostrils and apply protective ointment if the skin appears excoriated. Properly dispose of the gloves and wash your hands.

Oropharyngeal airway

A rubber or plastic device, an oropharyngeal airway is inserted through the mouth and into the posterior pharynx. Because the unconscious patient's tongue usually obstructs the posterior pharynx, this airway conforms to the curvature of the palate, correcting the obstruction and allowing air to pass around and through the tube.

Indications. An oropharyngeal airway is indicated to ease suctioning and provide short-term prevention or relief of soft-tissue upper airway obstruction in the unconscious patient.

Trauma to the lower face, recent oral surgery, or loose or avulsed teeth contraindicate the use of an oropharyngeal airway.

Insertion. First, select the appropriate-size airway for your patient — an oversize airway can obstruct breathing by depressing the epiglottis into the laryngeal opening. Usually you'll select a small size for an infant or child, a medium size for an average adult, and a large size for a large or obese adult. Confirm the correct size by placing the airway flange beside the patient's cheek, parallel to his front teeth. If the size is correct, the airway's curve should reach to the angle of the jaw.

Also, gather clean gloves and, if necessary, a tongue depressor. Then follow these steps:

• Explain the procedure to the patient, even though he may not appear alert. Wash your hands and put on the clean gloves. If the patient is wearing dentures, remove them to prevent further airway obstruction. If necessary, suction the patient.

• Place the patient in a supine position with his neck hyperextended, unless contraindicated.

• Insert the airway using the cross-finger or tongue-depressor technique.

To use the cross-finger technique, place your thumb on the patient's upper teeth and your index finger on his lower teeth, gently pushing his mouth open. Try to point the airway tip toward the cheek, and gently advance it. Then rotate the airway by sliding the tip back over the tongue's surface until it's pointing downward. Be careful not to push the tongue back with the airway.

To use the tongue-depressor technique, open the patient's mouth and depress his tongue with the blade. Guide the artificial airway over the back of the tongue, as in the cross-finger technique, until it's in place.

• Properly dispose of the gloves and wash your hands.

Routine care. Auscultate the patient's lungs to ensure adequate ventilation, and position the patient on his side to decrease the risk of vomitus aspiration.

Frequently check the airway for dislodgment and perform mouth care every 2 to 4 hours, as needed. To clean the airway, hold the patient's jaw open with a padded tongue depressor and remove the airway as described below. Then clean it as you would a nasopharyngeal airway, complete standard mouth care, and reinsert the airway.

Whenever you remove the airway to perform mouth care, check the mucous membranes of the mouth and the lips for ulceration and tissue damage, which can result from prolonged airway use. Always document the procedure and your care measures.

Complications. Inserting an oropharyngeal airway can damage or knock out the patient's teeth as well as cause tissue damage and bleeding. If these complications occur, remove the airway as described below and notify the doctor before reinserting it.

Removing the airway. Expect to remove the airway when the patient no longer needs it or when the airway needs cleaning. Evaluate the patient's behavior for signs that he no longer needs the airway. As he becomes more alert, for example, he's likely to cough or gag. When the patient regains consciousness and can swallow, the airway can safely be removed.

To remove an oropharyngeal airway, wash your hands, put on clean gloves, and pull the airway outward and downward, following the mouth's natural curves. Properly dispose of the airway and gloves, and wash your hands again.

After removing the airway, test the patient's cough and gag reflexes and auscultate his lungs to ensure that he no longer needs the artificial airway.

Endotracheal tube

Used for short-term ventilation, endotracheal intubation involves the nasal or oral insertion of a flexible, cuffed tube through the larynx and into the trachea. Only a doctor, respiratory therapist, or specially trained nurse can perform endotracheal intubation. It's used to relieve airway obstruction when all other efforts to maintain an open airway have failed. Endotracheal tubes can also be used to administer medication in an emergency.

Indications. Nasal endotracheal intubation is indicated when a patient has facial, oral, or cervical neck trauma or a jaw movement problem. A nasal endotracheal tube also provides a controlled airway for mechanical ventilation that's more comfortable than an oral endotracheal tube.

Contraindications include a nasal obstruction, a fractured nose, sinusitis, and bleeding disorders. A nasal endotracheal tube should be used cautiously in patients with basal skull fractures when communication exists between the nasopharyngeal mucosa and the brain.

Oral endotracheal intubation provides an open airway during cardiopulmonary resuscitation; it also offers a controlled airway for mechanical ventilation when the patient has a nasal obstruction or a predisposition to nosebleeds. This type of intubation is contraindicated for patients with trauma to the lower face or mouth and for those who've recently undergone oral surgery.

Both nasal and oral endotracheal tubes are contraindicated in patients with epiglottitis; acute, unstable cervical spine injury; or laryngeal obstruction caused by tumor, infection, or vocal cord paralysis. Tracheotomy remains the alternative treatment for such patients.

Preparing for intubation. To prepare for endotracheal tube insertion, first collect an intubation tray with the following equipment: an endotracheal tube and a spare tube in the same size; a 10-ml syringe; an oral airway or block for oral intubation; a light laryngoscope with a handle and different-size curved and straight blades; a sedative and a local anesthetic spray; sterile drape, towel, gloves, water, basin, and gauze sponge; water-soluble lubricant; adhesive tape; compound benzoin tincture; a stylet; Magill forceps; a stethoscope; a swivel adapter; suction equipment; a manual resuscitation bag, such as an Ambu bag; and equipment for administering humidified oxygen. You might not use all the equipment on the tray for the procedure.

Then follow these steps:
• If possible, explain the procedure to the patient to gain his cooperation and make insertion easier.
• Check the battery-operated light in the laryngoscope handle by snapping the appropriate-size blade in place for intubation. If the light fails to flash immediately, replace the laryngoscope bulb or the batteries, whichever is indicated.
• Open sterile packages. Squeeze water-soluble lubricant onto a sterile field.
• Attach the syringe to the port of the tube's exterior pilot cuff and inflate the cuff slowly, observing for uniform inflation. Check the cuff for leaks. Use the syringe to completely deflate the cuff.
• To ease insertion of a nasal endotracheal tube, lubricate the tube cover with water-soluble lubricant. You rarely use a lubricant for oral intubation.
• Lubricate the entire stylet, if necessary, so it can be easily removed from the tube after the procedure. Insert it so that its distal tip lies about ½″ (1.3 cm) inside the endotracheal tube's distal end. Prevent vocal cord trauma by making sure the stylet doesn't extend beyond the tube.
• Prepare the humidified oxygen system and the suctioning equipment for immediate use.

Insertion. This procedure covers oral endotracheal intubation only. If you're qualified to perform it, follow these steps:

• Check the doctor's written order and assess the patient's condition.
• Wash your hands and put on gloves.
• Administer medication to decrease respiratory secretions, induce amnesia or analgesia, and help calm and relax the conscious patient, as ordered. Remove any dentures.
• If necessary, suction the patient just before you insert the tube so you can visualize the pharyngeal and vocal cord structure. Use a tonsil suction tip to suction near the vocal cords if secretions cloud visualization.
• Place the patient in a supine position with his neck hyperextended to straighten the pharynx and trachea.
• Spray a local anesthetic into the posterior pharynx to help quell the patient's gag reflex and to reduce his discomfort during intubation.
• Hyperoxygenate the patient, using a manual resuscitation bag with a face mask attached to an oxygen source and the flowmeter set at 15 liters/minute for 1 to 2 minutes.
• Grasp the laryngoscope handle in your dominant hand and gently slide the blade into the right side of the patient's mouth. Then center the blade, pushing the tongue to the left. Hold the lower lip away from the teeth to prevent injury.
• Advance the blade, bringing the handle toward you to expose the epiglottis. Avoid using the patient's teeth as a pivotal point for the laryngoscope because this may damage them.
• Continue to lift the laryngoscope handle toward you to reveal the vocal cords. With the vocal cords in view, guide the endotracheal tube into the right side of the mouth and down along the laryngoscope blade into the vertical larynx opening between the vocal cords. Don't mis-

take the horizontal esophageal opening for the larynx. If the vocal cords are closed in spasm, wait a few seconds for them to relax, then guide the tube gently past them.
• Advance the tube until the cuff disappears beyond the vocal cords. Further insertion may occlude a major bronchus and cause lung collapse.
• Holding the endotracheal tube in place, quickly remove the stylet.
• Inflate the tube cuff until you feel resistance. Once you've finished the procedure, use either the minimal leak or minimal occlusive volume technique to establish correct cuff inflation.

To perform the minimal leak technique, attach a 10-ml syringe to the port on the tube's exterior pilot cuff and place a stethoscope on the side of the patient's neck. Inject small amounts of air during the inspiratory phase of ventilation until you can't hear a leak. Then aspirate 0.1 cc of air from the cuff to create a minimal air leak. To perform the minimal occlusive volume technique, follow the first two steps of the minimal leak technique, placing your stethoscope over the trachea instead of the side of the neck. Then aspirate until you hear a small leak on inspiration, and add just enough air to stop the leak. Record the amount of air needed to inflate the cuff for subsequent monitoring for tracheal dilation or erosion.
• Feel the tube's tip for warm exhalation and listen for air movement to ensure proper placement. If the patient breathes spontaneously, observe for chest expansion and auscultate the chest for bilateral breath sounds. If he's unconscious or uncooperative, use a manual resuscitation bag and observe for upper chest movement. If his stomach distends and belching occurs,

the tube is in the esophagus. Immediately deflate the cuff, remove the tube, and repeat insertion, using another sterile tube.
• If you don't hear breath sounds on both sides of the chest, you may have inserted the tube into a main-stem bronchus (usually the right one, because it's more vertical than the left and has a wider angle at the bifurcation). Such an insertion occludes the other bronchus and lung and results in atelectasis on the obstructed side. If the tube rests on the carina, the patient will cough and fight the ventilator. To correct these problems, deflate the cuff, withdraw the tube ½" to 1" (1.3 to 2.5 cm), auscultate for bilateral breath sounds, and reinflate the cuff.
• After you've confirmed correct tube placement, administer oxygen or initiate mechanical ventilation, and provide suction, as needed.
• Secure the tube, taking care not to catch the patient's lips in the tape.
• Inflate the cuff, using either the minimal leak or minimal occlusive volume technique described above.
• Note the tube's exit point by recording the centimeter reading at the corner of the mouth. If the tube doesn't have centimeter marks, clearly mark the exit point with a water-resistant pen or tape. Periodic monitoring of this mark can reveal tube displacement.
• Ensure that a chest X-ray is taken to verify the tube's position.
• Place a swivel adapter between the tube and the humidified oxygen source to allow for intermittent suctioning and to reduce tension on the tube.
• Properly dispose of the gloves and wash your hands.

Routine care. After the tube has been inserted, place the patient with his head in a comfortable position to avoid tube kinking and airway obstruction. Auscultate both sides of the anterior chest and check chest movement hourly to ensure correct tube placement and full lung ventilation. Give frequent oral care and reposition the endotracheal tube every 8 hours to avoid pressure sores on the sides of the mouth.

• *Suctioning.* When necessary, suction the endotracheal tube to keep it clear from secretions and mucus plugs (see *Suctioning an endotracheal or tracheostomy tube.*) By keeping the patient's airway patent, suctioning promotes optimal gas exchange and prevents the pneumonia that results from collected secretions. But if suctioning is performed incorrectly, it can cause serious complications, including hypoxia, infection, and life-threatening arrhythmias. You can help reduce the risk of complications by following these tips:

• Hyperinflate and oxygenate the patient's lungs before and after suctioning.

• Maintain sterile technique.

• Complete the task quickly.

• Apply suction for no more than 10 seconds.

• Closely monitor the patient's vital signs.

Perform suctioning cautiously in patients who've recently had a tracheotomy or other tracheal or upper respiratory surgery, patients with blood dyscrasias, and patients receiving anticoagulant therapy, which may make bleeding more likely.

If the patient is on mechanical ventilation or positive end-expiratory pressure, you may use closed tracheal suctioning to prevent the disruption of therapy and the temporary decrease in oxygen that occur with conventional suctioning.

• *Securing the tube.* Each time you assess the patient, make sure his endotracheal tube is taped securely. Retape as necessary.

Before taping a tube in place, make sure the patient's face is clean, dry, and free of beard stubble. If possible, suction his mouth and dry the endotracheal tube just before taping. After taping, always check for bilateral breath sounds to make sure the tube hasn't been displaced by manipulation. To secure an endotracheal tube, you can use one of three techniques.

To use the first method, follow these steps:

• Cut two 2″ (5-cm) strips and two 15″ (38-cm) strips of 1″ cloth adhesive tape. Then cut a 13″ (33-cm) slit in one end of each 15″ strip.

• Apply compound benzoin tincture to the patient's cheeks. Don't spray it directly on the face because the vapors can be irritating if they are inhaled or get in the eyes. Instead, spray the benzoin on a gauze pad and wipe the patient's cheeks.

• Place a 2″ strip on each of the patient's cheeks. This creates a new surface on which to anchor the tape that secures the endotracheal tube and helps preserve skin integrity if frequent retaping becomes necessary. If the patient's skin appears excoriated or at risk, protect it with transparent dressing.

• Apply compound benzoin tincture to the tape on the patient's face and to the part of the tube where you'll be applying tape to anchor it.

• On the side of the mouth where the tube will be anchored, place the unslit end of the 15″ strip of tape on top of the tape on the patient's cheek. Just before taping, check the reference mark on the tube to ensure correct placement.

• Wrap the top half of the tape

(Text continues on page 92.)

Suctioning an endotracheal or tracheostomy tube

To suction an endotracheal or a tracheostomy tube, follow these steps.

Gather supplies
Wash your hands and gather sterile saline solution, a sterile gown and mask, a clean glove, and a suction kit containing a wrapper that you'll use as your sterile field, a sterile suction catheter (usually #12 or #14 French), a sterile cup for saline solution, and one sterile glove. (Most kits contain only one glove, but you'll need two—one sterile and one clean.)

At the patient's bedside, you'll need an oxygen flowmeter and suction apparatus, including a regulator, connecting tubing, and a collection bottle. You'll also need a plastic bag to dispose of the used supplies.

If you're working with an assistant, you'll also need a manual resuscitation bag with an adapter to provide 100% oxygen. If you're working alone, use the manual sigh settings on the ventilator.

Prepare the patient
Ensure privacy and explain the procedure to the patient, even if he's unresponsive. Auscultate his breath sounds and check his heart rate and rhythm.

Set up the equipment
Attach the connecting tubing to the suction collection bottle. Then pinch the connecting tubing and set the negative pressure regulator to approximately 120 mm Hg.

Next, open the suction kit by pulling the edges away from each other, being careful not to contaminate the inside of the wrapper, as shown at the top of the next column.

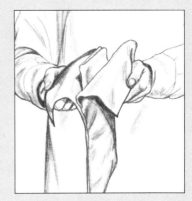

Spread the wrapper on the bedside table to serve as your sterile field. Maintaining sterile technique, put on the gloves. Your dominant hand will remain sterile; you'll use your nondominant hand for clean tasks.

With your sterile hand, set up the disposable, plastic-lined cardboard cup on the sterile field. With your nonsterile hand, pour sterile saline solution into the cup. You'll use this saline solution to rinse the catheter and check its patency.

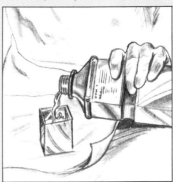

(continued)

Suctioning an endotracheal or tracheostomy tube *(continued)*

With your sterile hand, pull the catheter out of its wrapper, maintaining its sterility. Wrap the catheter around your sterile hand to reduce the risk of contamination. Hold the connecting tubing with your nonsterile hand and attach the catheter to the tubing.

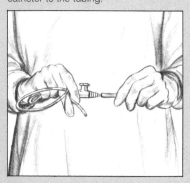

Check the pressure reading
With your sterile hand, pinch the catheter. Apply suction by placing the thumb of your nonsterile hand over the suction port.

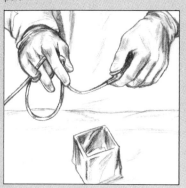

Check the reading on the suction regulator; it should be between 80 and 120 mm Hg. Adjust the suction pressure accordingly with your nonsterile hand.

Administer oxygen
Before suctioning, have your assistant hyperinflate the patient's lungs and give him extra oxygen with the manual resuscitation bag.

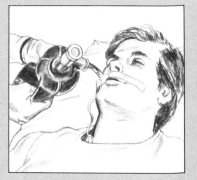

If you aren't working with an assistant, use the manual sigh settings on the ventilator. Make sure they're set correctly and the oxygen concentration setting is at 100%.

Check catheter patency
Place the end of the catheter in the sterile saline solution and then apply suction, drawing up the solution until it reaches the collection bottle. This allows you to check the catheter patency and the effectiveness of suctioning, as well as lubricate the catheter.

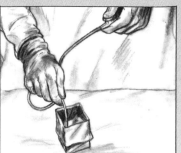

Apply suction

Warn the patient that he may feel short of breath, then gently advance the catheter through the endotracheal tube. To avoid damaging the mucosa, don't apply suction or jab the catheter up and down while it advances. Stop advancing the catheter when it reaches the carina (you'll feel resistance, and usually the patient will cough).

Withdraw the catheter about 1 cm from the carina and then suction. While suctioning, rotate the catheter gently and withdraw it in one continuous motion. Don't apply suction for longer than 10 seconds.

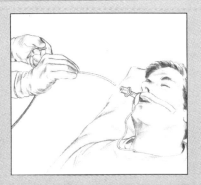

From catheter insertion to withdrawal, the whole procedure should take no more than 10 seconds.

If you need to suction the tube further, rinse the catheter in the sterile saline solution and repeat the procedure.

Reconnect the ventilator

When you've finished suctioning and the patient has received enough oxygen, reconnect the ventilator tubing to the endotracheal tube, if necessary. If you used the manual sigh settings on the ventilator, return the controls to their original settings. After rinsing the catheter, suction the patient's mouth and pharynx to remove any excess saliva and oropharyngeal secretions.

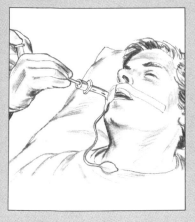

Withdraw the catheter

Completely remove the catheter as shown at the top of the next column. Then have your assistant reconnect the manual resuscitation bag to give the patient some deep, oxygen-rich breaths. Or use the manual sigh mechanism on the ventilator if you're working alone. Assess for dyspnea and discomfort. If the patient is connected to a cardiac monitor, check his heart rhythm.

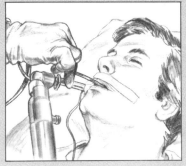

(continued)

Suctioning an endotracheal or tracheostomy tube *(continued)*

Assess the patient's breath sounds, and heart rate and rhythm. Then compare these findings with the baseline values.

Dispose of materials

Remove the catheter from the connecting tubing after rinsing again. Now wrap the catheter around the fingers of your sterile hand and pull the sterile glove off so the catheter remains inside, as shown.

Place the catheter and glove inside

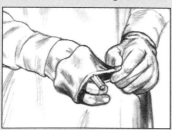

the plastic bag and follow any special isolation procedures for contaminated materials. Next, remove the other glove and mask.

Discard the saline solution. Fold the sterile field over the used supplies and put it in the plastic bag. Discard the bag according to hospital procedure. Next, wash your hands and restock any supplies at the bedside as necessary.

Document care

Document the procedure and your assessment findings before and after suctioning. Record the color, consistency, and amount of secretions (in milliliters). Also note any adverse reactions to suctioning and the steps you took to alleviate them.

around the tube twice, pulling the tape as lightly as possible. Then, directing the tape over the patient's upper lip, place the end of it on the patient's other cheek. Cut off any excess tape.
• Use the lower half of the tape to secure an oral airway if necessary. Or twist the lower half of the tape around the tube twice and attach it to the original cheek. Taping in opposite directions places equal traction on the tube.
• If you've taped an oral airway or are concerned about the stability, apply the other 15″ strip of tape in the same manner as the first, starting on the other side of the patient's face. If the tape around the tube feels too bulky, use only the upper part of the tape and cut off the

lower part. If copious oral secretions are present, seal the tape by placing a 1″ (2.5-cm) piece of benzoin-sealed paper tape over the adhesive tape.

To use the second method, follow these steps:
• Cut one piece of 1″ cloth adhesive tape long enough to wrap around the patient's head and overlap in front. Then, cut an 8″ (20-cm) piece of tape and center it on the longer piece, sticky sides together. Next, cut a 5″ (12.5-cm) slit in each end.
• Apply compound benzoin tincture to the patient's cheeks and under his nose, again applying it indirectly to the face.
• Place the top half of one end of the tape under the patient's nose and

wrap the lower half around the endotracheal tube. Place the lower half of the other end of the tape under the patient's nose and wrap the top half around the tube.

To use the third method, follow these steps:

• Cut a tracheostomy tie in two pieces (one a few inches longer than the other), and cut two 6" (15-cm) pieces of 1" cloth adhesive tape. Next, cut a 2" (5-cm) slit in one end of both pieces of tape. Fold the other end of the tape so that the sticky sides are together, and cut a small hole in it.

• Apply compound benzoin tincture to the part of the endotracheal tube that will be taped.

• Wrap the slit ends of each piece of tape around the tube — one piece on each side. To secure the tape, overlap it.

• Apply the free ends of the tape to both sides of the patient's face. Then insert the tracheostomy ties through the holes in the ends of the tape and knot the ties.

• Bring the longer tie behind the patient's neck and tie it to the shorter tie at one side of his neck. Knotting on the side prevents the patient from lying on the knot and getting a pressure sore.

• *Checking cuff pressure.* Regardless of the cuff design or inflation technique used, monitor cuff pressure once every 4 to 8 hours. (See *How to measure tracheal cuff pressure,* pages 94 and 95.)

Keep the intubation equipment accessible in case accidental extubation occurs. Thoroughly document the procedure and your care measures.

Complications. Potential complications of endotracheal intubation include apnea caused by reflex breath-holding; bronchospasm; aspi-

ration of blood, secretions, or gastric contents; tooth damage or loss; trauma to the lips, mouth, pharynx, or larynx (vocal cord damage); laryngeal edema and erosion; and tracheal stenosis, erosion, and necrosis.

These complications relate directly to the size of the tube, duration of intubation, cuff pressure, and amount of tube movement. They can be prevented by using the proper-size tube, by using a tracheostomy tube to protect the vocal cords when long-term intubation is necessary, by using a swivel adapter, and by suctioning and retaping the tube only when necessary. Also, instruct the patient not to mouth words, because the vocal cords move by reflex and press against the endotracheal tube. Finally, decrease the patient's head movement as much as possible.

If apnea occurs, use a manual resuscitation bag to artificially breathe for the patient. If aspiration occurs, suction the airway until it clears, notify the doctor, and monitor for signs of infection. If you detect stridor, dyspnea, or any other sign of tissue damage, notify the doctor at once.

Removing the tube. To remove the endotracheal tube, follow these steps:

• Wash your hands and put on gloves. Explain the procedure to the patient.

• Elevate the head of the patient's bed to approximately 90 degrees. Suction the secretions inside and outside the tube.

• Attach a 10-ml syringe to the pilot balloon port, and aspirate air until you meet resistance and the pilot balloon deflates. *Never cut the pilot balloon to deflate the cuff.*

(Text continues on page 96.)

How to measure tracheal cuff pressure

An endotracheal or tracheostomy cuff provides a closed system for mechanical ventilation so the desired tidal volume can be delivered to the patient's lungs. It also protects the patient's lower respiratory tract from secretions or gastric contents that may accumulate in the pharynx.

To perform these functions, the cuff must exert enough pressure on the tracheal wall to seal the airway. Excessive pressure, however, can compromise arterial, capillary, or venous flow to the tracheal mucosa.

Measuring cuff pressure
The ideal cuff pressure is the lowest amount needed to seal the airway—known as minimal occlusive volume (MOV). Many authorities recommend maintaining a cuff pressure lower than venous perfusion pressure—usually about 18 mm Hg. Although that's a good guideline, the actual cuff pressure level you'll want to maintain will vary with each patient. To ensure your patient's cuff pressure remains within safe limits, measure MOV at least once a shift.

Preparing for the procedure
Before the procedure, gather a three-way stopcock, a 10-ml syringe partially filled with air, a mercury manometer, and suction equipment.

Then suction the endotracheal tube and the patient's oropharynx to remove secretions that have accumulated above the cuff.

Performing the procedure
Connect the ports of the three-way stopcock to the manometer tubing, the syringe, and the pilot balloon of the cuff. Close the port to the pilot balloon so air can't escape from the cuff.

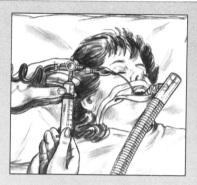

Instill air from the syringe into the manometer tubing until the pressure reading reaches 10 mm Hg. (When you open the stopcock to the cuff and the manometer, this air will prevent sudden cuff deflation.)

Turn off the stopcock to the syringe. Then record the manometer reading on expiration; this is the cuff pressure at MOV. (The mercury level will fluctuate as the patient inhales and exhales.) If cuff pressure is less than 25 mm Hg, turn off the stopcock to the pilot balloon.

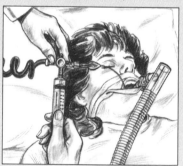

Rechecking MOV
If cuff pressure exceeds 25 mm Hg, double-check your reading. Turn off the

stopcock to the manometer and deflate the cuff completely.

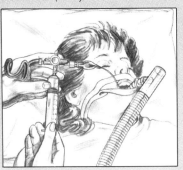

Reinflate the cuff until you no longer hear an air leak on inspiration. (Airways are larger on inspiration than on expiration, so if you stop reinflating the cuff when you no longer hear a leak on expiration, a leak may still occur on inspiration.)

Auscultate the patient's trachea. A smooth, hollow sound indicates a sealed airway; a loud, gurgling sound indicates an air leak.

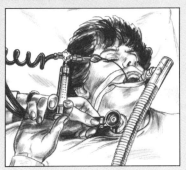

If you hear an air leak on inspiration, add air to the cuff in 0.1-ml increments until you can't hear the leak. Then remove air from the cuff until you can aus-cultate a small leak on inspiration, and add just enough air to stop the leak. Repeat the steps you took above to record the manometer reading on expiration. Then turn off the stopcock to the pilot balloon and disconnect the stopcock as shown.

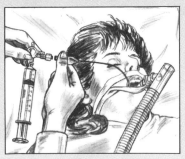

If the cuff pressure still exceeds 25 mm Hg, notify the doctor. Document your findings.

A patient with a high airway pressure or positive end-expiratory pressure may need an extremely high cuff pressure to seal the airway. Ask the doctor if the patient can tolerate such a high cuff pressure or a minimal leak in the cuff, or if he should be reintubated. Then document the decision and the reasons behind it.

If the tube is too small, you may not be able to seal the airway without over-inflating the cuff. Report this to the doctor, because the tube may need to be replaced with a larger one.

Record the amount of air needed for reinflation. A gradual increase in the amount needed to reach MOV may indicate tracheal malacia (an abnormal softening of the tracheal tissue). But maintaining cuff pressure at the lowest possible level and inflating it to MOV will keep cuff-related complications to a minimum.

• Hyperinflate the patient's lungs for 1 minute with a manual resuscitation bag attached to an oxygen source with the flowmeter set at 15 liters/minute. Or use the manual sigh mechanism on a mechanical ventilator with 100% oxygen. This will increase his oxygen reserve and let you detect air leaks around the deflated cuff. If you fail to detect a leak, notify the doctor immediately and don't proceed with extubation. Absence of an air leak may indicate marked tracheal edema and can result in total airway obstruction when you remove the endotracheal tube.

• If you detect the proper air leak, untape the endotracheal tube while another nurse holds it.

• Insert a sterile suction catheter through the endotracheal tube, apply suction, and ask the patient to open his mouth fully and pretend to cry out. This causes vocal cord abduction and reduces the risk of laryngeal trauma during tube withdrawal.

• Simultaneously remove the endotracheal tube and the suction catheter in one smooth outward and downward motion, following the natural curve of the patient's mouth. Suctioning during extubation removes secretions retained at the end of the tube and prevents aspiration of those secretions.

Alternatively, ask another nurse to deliver a large breath with a manual resuscitation bag, keeping the bag compressed for 2 to 3 seconds. Remove the tube and the catheter just as the other nurse releases the resuscitation bag. The forced expiratory gas flow will carry secretions out of the central airways, helping the patient to expectorate them.

• Provide humidified supplemental oxygen, as ordered. Tell the patient to take 6 to 10 deep breaths. Monitor his respiratory status closely, and be prepared to reintubate if necessary.

• Properly dispose of the endotracheal tube and the gloves, and wash your hands.

Tracheostomy tube

Created surgically, a tracheostomy is an external opening to the trachea. An indwelling tube inserted into the tracheostomy prevents the opening from closing. This procedure minimizes the risk of vocal cord damage from an endotracheal tube during long-term airway support. It also maintains airway patency and skin and mucous membrane integrity, and prevents infection.

Metal and plastic tracheostomy tubes come in various sizes to accommodate patients of all ages. A metal or plastic uncuffed tube usually has three parts: an outer cannula, an inner cannula, and an obturator that serves as a guide for outer cannula insertion. Many plastic tubes consist simply of the obturator and one single-walled tube. Unlike a metal tube, a plastic tube doesn't require removal for cleaning because encrustations are less likely to form on nonmetal materials. (See *Comparing tracheostomy tubes.*)

Indications. A tracheotomy is indicated when a patient has complete upper airway obstruction and when endotracheal intubation is impossible. Usually preferred for long-term intubation, it can also be used to provide airway access in a patient with unmanageable secretions.

Routine care. After the doctor performs the tracheotomy, you'll provide routine care of the tracheos-

Comparing tracheostomy tubes

Made of either plastic or metal, tracheostomy tubes come in uncuffed, cuffed, and fenestrated varieties. Tube selection depends on the patient's condition and the doctor's preference. The following chart lists the advantages and disadvantages of some commonly used tubes.

TYPE	ADVANTAGES	DISADVANTAGES
Uncuffed (plastic or metal)	• Permits free flow of air around the tube and through the larynx • Reduces risk of tracheal damage • Doesn't require a cuff, making it a good choice for children	• Increases the risk of aspiration in adults because of the absence of a cuff • May require adapter for mechanical ventilation
Cuffed (plastic; low pressure and high volume)	• Disposable • Won't detach accidentally inside the trachea because the cuff is bonded to the tube • Doesn't require periodic deflating to lower pressure because the cuff pressure is low and evenly distributed against the tracheal wall • Reduces the risk of tracheal damage	• May be costlier than other tubes
Fenestrated (plastic)	• Permits speech through the upper airway when the external opening is capped and the cuff is deflated • Allows breathing by mechanical ventilation with inner cannula in place and cuff inflated • Allows easy removal of the inner cannula for cleaning	• Fenestrations may become occluded • May allow the inner cannula to become dislodged

tomy tube and the stoma, usually using strict sterile technique to prevent infection. Some evidence suggests that you can perform safe care using clean technique. This care consists of cleaning the tube and the site. Expect to provide such care as often as every 30 minutes immediately after the tracheotomy and then once a shift. You'll also suction the patient before giving routine care and as necessary during your shift. The tracheostomy ties should be changed daily or as necessary.

• *Preparing for routine care.* Before performing routine care measures, assemble the equipment and supplies you'll need, including a waterproof trash bag; two sterile containers; sterile saline solution; hydrogen peroxide; a hemostat; bandage scissors; and sterile gloves, cotton-tipped applicators, and 4″ × 4″ gauze sponges or prepackaged sterile tracheostomy dressing. You'll also need equipment for suctioning, mouth care, cuff procedures, and changing the tracheostomy ties.

After you've gathered the equipment, explain the procedures to the patient, even if he's unresponsive. Then wash your hands and follow these steps:

• Place the cuffed trash bag next to your work area.

• Establish a sterile field near the patient's bed and place sterile equipment and supplies on it.

• Pour the sterile solutions into the sterile containers.

• Prepare new tracheostomy ties from twill tape, if indicated.

• If using a spare sterile inner cannula, unscrew the cap from the top of the sterile container, but don't remove it.

• Assess the patient's condition. Unless contraindicated, place him in semi-Fowler's position.

• Remove any humidification or ventilation device.

• Using sterile technique, suction the entire length of the tracheostomy tube to remove any secretions.

• Reconnect the patient to the humidifier or ventilator if necessary.

• Remove and discard the patient's tracheostomy dressing.

• *Cleaning a single-cannula tube.* If your patient has a single-cannula tube, clean it by following these steps:

• Put a sterile glove on your dominant hand.

• With your gloved hand, wet a sterile 4″ × 4″ gauze sponge with hydrogen peroxide solution and saline solution for cleaning. Squeeze out excess liquid to prevent accidental aspiration. Then wipe the patient's neck under the tracheostomy tube flanges and twill tapes.

• Saturate a second sponge and wipe clean the skin surrounding the tracheostomy. Use additional sponges or cotton-tipped applicators to clean the stoma site and the tube flanges. Wipe from the stoma outward only once with each sponge and then discard it.

• Remove encrustations with a sterile cotton-tipped applicator saturated with hydrogen peroxide. (Be sure you press out the excess liquid before wiping the site.) Wipe gently, especially if the surrounding skin appears excoriated. Use each applicator only once.

• Rinse debris and any hydrogen peroxide with one or more sterile 4″ × 4″ gauze sponges dampened in sterile saline solution. Dry the area thoroughly with additional sterile gauze sponges. Remove and discard the glove.

• *Cleaning a double-cannula tube.* If your patient has a double-cannula tube, you'll need to gather additional equipment, including a sterile nylon brush; sterile 6″ (15-cm) pipe cleaners; a third sterile solution container; a clean glove; a spare inner cannula for a patient on a ventilator; and, possibly, an additional basin to hold your gauze sponges and cotton-tipped applicators saturated with cleaning solution. Then clean the tube by following these steps:

• Put a sterile glove on your dominant hand and a clean glove on your nondominant hand.

• With your nondominant hand, disconnect the ventilator or humidification device. Then, with your dominant hand, unlock and remove the tracheostomy tube's inner cannula.

• Soak the inner cannula in the container of hydrogen peroxide to remove encrustations.

• If the patient is on a mechanical ventilator and can't tolerate being disconnected, use your nondominant hand to remove the lid from the container with the spare inner cannula. Pick up the cannula with your dominant hand and insert it into the outer cannula of the patient's tracheostomy tube. Use your nondominant hand to reconnect the patient to the ventilator. For these patients, perform tracheostomy care and apply a new sterile dressing as described below *before* cleaning the inner cannula. After you've cleaned the inner cannula, it will become the patient's new spare.

• Use your dominant hand to clean the skin, stoma, and tracheostomy tube flanges with the presoaked gauze sponges and cotton-tipped applicators, as described above.

• Pick up the inner cannula from the soaking container and scrub it with the nylon brush. If the brush doesn't slide in easily, use a pipe cleaner.

• Immerse the cannula in the container of saline solution and agitate

it for about 10 seconds. This rinses it and provides a thin film of lubrication to ease replacement.

• Hold the cannula up to the light to see if it's clean. If you still see encrustations, repeat the cleaning process. If it's clean, tap the cannula gently against the inside edge of the sterile container to remove excess liquid, preventing possible aspiration. Use three pipe cleaners twisted together to dry the inside of the catheter. Don't dry the outer surface because you'll remove the lubricating film.

• Gently reinsert the inner cannula into the patient's tracheostomy tube. Lock it in place and pull on it gently to ensure its secure positioning.

• Apply a new sterile tracheostomy dressing. If you're not using a commercially prepared dressing, don't select cotton-filled gauze or a trimmed gauze sponge because the lint and fibers can be aspirated and cause a tracheal abscess. Instead, open a sterile 4″ × 4″ gauze pad to its full length and fold it in half lengthwise to form a long, thin rectangle. With the folded edge facing downward, find the center of the edge; then fold each side straight up from this point to create a U-shaped pad. Slip the pad under the flanges of the tracheostomy tube so that the pad's flaps encircle and cushion the tube.

• *Replacing the ties.* You shouldn't change the tracheostomy ties during the immediate postoperative period unless necessary. This gives the stoma a chance to form (a process that usually takes 4 days) and helps prevent accidental dislodgment and tube expulsion. After that, change the ties daily or as necessary by following these steps:

• Because the patient's movement or coughing may dislodge the tube during this procedure, enlist the aid of another nurse or a respiratory therapist.

• If you're not using commercially packaged tracheostomy ties, prepare new ties from a 30″ (76-cm) length of twill tape by folding one end back 1″ (2.5 cm) on itself. Then, with bandage scissors, cut a ½″ (1.3-cm) slit down the center of the tape from the folded edge. Or you may fold the end of the tape and cut a small hole at each end of the tie.

• Prepare the other end of the tape in the same manner.

• Hold both ends together and cut the tape so that one piece is about 10″ (25 cm) long and the other is about 20″ (50 cm) long.

• After your assistant puts on sterile gloves, have her hold the tracheostomy tube in place. If you have to perform the procedure alone, prevent tube expulsion by fastening the clean ties in place before removing the old ones.

• While your assistant holds the tracheostomy tube, cut the soiled tracheostomy ties or untie and discard them. Before cutting, be sure that the pilot balloon for the tube cuff isn't in the path of the scissors.

• Working from the underside, thread the slit end of one new tie a short distance through the eye of one tracheostomy tube flange. If necessary, use the hemostat to pull the tie through. Then thread the other end of the tie completely through the slit end and pull it taut so that it loops firmly through the tube's flange. This avoids knots that can cause discomfort and lead to throat tissue irritation, pressure, and necrosis.

• Fasten the second tie to the opposite flange in the same manner.

• Instruct the patient to flex his neck while you bring the ties around his neck to the side and tie them together. Flexion produces the same neck circumference as coughing and helps prevent a connection that's too tight. As you tie, have your assistant place one finger under the tapes to ensure the ties are tight enough to avoid slippage, but loose enough to prevent choking or jugular vein constriction. Placing the closure on the side allows easy access and prevents pressure necrosis at the back of the neck when the patient reclines.

• After securing the ties, cut off the excess tape and instruct your assistant to release the tracheostomy tube.

• *Completing your care.* After you've replaced the tracheostomy ties, follow these steps:

• Replace any humidification device.

• Provide oral care as needed. The patient's mouth may become dry and malodorous and develop sores from encrusted secretions.

• Dispose of the gloves properly and then wash your hands.

• Make sure the patient is comfortable and can easily reach his call signal and communication aids.

• Examine the soiled dressings for the amount, color, consistency, and odor of drainage.

Nursing considerations. Don't change a single-cannula tracheostomy tube or the outer cannula of a double-cannula tube. Because of the risk of tracheal complications, the doctor will change the tube only when necessary.

If the patient will be discharged with a tracheostomy, begin teaching him home care procedures (using clean technique) as soon as he appears receptive. If he's going home with suction equipment, make sure he and his family know how to use the equipment.

Measure tracheal cuff pressure every 4 to 8 hours to prevent tracheal dilation, necrosis, and stenosis. If the patient's neck or stoma looks excoriated or infected, apply a water-soluble topical lubricant or antibiotic cream, as ordered. Remember not to use a powder or an oil-based substance on or around a stoma because aspiration can cause infection and abscess.

According to hospital policy, regularly replace all equipment, including solutions, to reduce the risk of nosocomial infections.

Complications. Within the first 48 hours after tracheostomy tube insertion — and occasionally even later — the following complications may occur: hemorrhage at the operative site, causing drowning; bleeding or edema within tracheal tissues, causing airway obstruction; aspiration of secretions, resulting in pneumonia; introduction of air into the pleural cavity, causing pneumothorax; hypoxia, acidosis, or sudden electrolyte shifts, triggering cardiac arrest; and introduction of air into surrounding tissues, causing subcutaneous emphysema.

After the first 48 hours, infection at the stoma or any site distal to it can lead to pneumonia from aspirated secretions. Also, secretions may collect under dressings and twill tape, producing skin excoriation and infection. Hardened mucus or a slipped cuff on a metal tube can occlude the cannula opening and obstruct the airway. Tube displacement can cause blood vessel erosion and hemorrhage. Tracheal erosion and necrosis can result from the tube's presence or cuff pressure.

Always have the following emergency equipment ready and in full view in the patient's room: suctioning equipment and supplies,

because the patient may need his airway cleared at any time; a manual resuscitation bag attached to oxygen; the sterile obturator originally used to insert the patient's tracheostomy tube, for quick reinsertion upon tube expulsion; another sterile tracheostomy tube (with obturator) the same size as the one in use, to replace a contaminated or expelled tube; and a spare sterile inner cannula to replace a contaminated or expelled inner cannula.

Optional emergency equipment includes a sterile tracheostomy tube (with obturator) one size smaller than the one in use, to replace an expelled tube when the trachea immediately begins to close (this makes insertion of a tube of the original size difficult); and a sterile tracheal dilator or sterile hemostat to maintain an open airway before you insert a new tracheostomy tube. Always follow hospital policy regarding tracheostomy emergency procedures. (See *Emergency management: Obstructed tracheostomy tube,* page 102.)

Bronchoscopy
When an obstruction occurs in the more distal airways, a doctor may perform bronchoscopy. He'll use a metal or fiber-optic bronchoscope, which allows direct visualization of the trachea and tracheobronchial tree through a slender, flexible tube with mirrors and a light at its distal end. If necessary, biopsy forceps, a brush, or a catheter may be passed through the bronchoscope to obtain specimens for cytologic and bacteriologic examinations.

Most often, doctors use a flexible fiber-optic bronchoscope because it's smaller, allows a greater viewing range of the segmental and subsegmental bronchi, and carries less risk of trauma than a rigid metal

PROCEDURES

Emergency management: Obstructed tracheostomy tube

If your patient has a tracheostomy, be prepared to handle common emergencies, such as an airway obstruction, which can occur any time after placement. One cause of a partial or complete obstruction is dry mucus secretions in the inner lumen of the tracheostomy tube.

Assessment
Suspect tube obstruction by a mucus plug if the patient appears pale and diaphoretic, and if you hear a whistling sound with each breath. His labored respirations will be rapid and shallow, and you'll feel minimal airflow at the stoma. He may look cyanotic.

If you hear a whistling sound and feel minimal airflow, you know he's receiving some air, but you must act quickly to remove the plug before he develops further respiratory distress.

Intervention
Call for assistance as you help the patient sit upright. Remove the tube's inner cannula and have him try to cough out the plug. (This may be difficult because he won't be able to perform Valsalva's maneuver or cough with an effective force.)

If this doesn't work, quickly attach a manual resuscitation bag with supplemental oxygen to his tracheostomy tube and deliver several vigorous hyperinflations. If they don't dislodge the plug or if you feel resistance to inflation, you'll need to suction. Prepare a syringe of 2 ml sterile isotonic saline solution (without preservatives). Instill the solution and vigorously suction for no longer than 10 seconds at a time. Hyperinflate with the supplemental oxygen between each suctioning attempt.

If you still haven't been able to establish an effective airway, call the doctor immediately, cut the tracheostomy ties, and gently remove the entire tube. Keep the stoma open with a Kelly clamp and try to insert a new tube. If you can't get the tube in, insert a suction catheter instead, and thread the tube over the catheter.

If you still can't establish an effective airway and you no longer detect a pulse, call a code. Then either ventilate with a face mask and resuscitation bag, or remove the Kelly clamp to close the stoma and perform mouth-to-mouth resuscitation until the doctor arrives. If air leaks from the stoma, cover it with an occlusive dressing. (Remember, don't leave this patient alone until you have established that he has an effective airway and can breathe comfortably.)

Once the patient has a new tracheostomy tube in place and can breathe more easily, provide supplemental humidified oxygen until he receives a full evaluation. Monitor his vital signs, skin color, and level of consciousness, and, unless contraindicated, elevate the head of his bed.

Prevention
Help prevent future episodes by monitoring the patient for tenacious, blood-tinged tracheal mucus, the telltale whistling sound, and decreased airflow at the stoma during respirations.

Keep his secretions liquefied by ensuring that he's well hydrated and that any oxygen received is humidified. If he's not receiving oxygen, use an ultrasonic humidifier.

Have the patient routinely perform coughing and deep-breathing exercises to mobilize secretions and facilitate expectoration. If that doesn't mobilize secretions, you can try routine chest physiotherapy.

bronchoscope. Doctors use a rigid bronchoscope to remove foreign objects, excise endobronchial lesions, and control massive hemoptysis.

Indications. Bronchoscopy is indicated to remove foreign bodies, cancerous or benign tumors, mucus plugs, or excessive secretions from the tracheobronchial tree. It's also indicated when the doctor wants to make a visual examination of a suspected tumor, obstruction, secretion, or foreign body in the tracheobronchial tree, as demonstrated on radiography. When used to obtain a specimen for bacteriologic or cytologic examination, bronchoscopy aids in diagnosing bronchogenic carcinoma, tuberculosis, interstitial pulmonary disease, and fungal or parasitic pulmonary infection. And it can be used to locate a bleeding site in the tracheobronchial tree.

Preparing for bronchoscopy. Prepare the patient for bronchoscopy by describing the procedure to him. If he has an obstruction, tell him he can expect relief immediately after the procedure.

Tell the patient that he may receive an intravenous sedative to help him relax. For children and extremely apprehensive adults, a general anesthetic may be administered in the operating room. If the patient won't be receiving a general anesthetic, inform him that a local anesthetic will be sprayed into his nose and mouth to suppress the gag reflex. He may also receive an aerosolized anesthetic via nebulizer before the procedure. Warn him that the spray has an unpleasant taste and that he can expect some discomfort and a feeling of breathlessness during the procedure. Reassure him that his airway

won't be blocked and he'll receive oxygen through the bronchoscope.

Make sure the patient or an appropriate family member has signed a consent form.

Before the procedure, check the patient's history for hypersensitivity to the anesthetic, and obtain baseline vital signs and arterial blood gas analysis. Administer a preoperative sedative, as ordered, and check his vital signs again. If the patient wears dentures, instruct him to remove them just before the procedure. Monitor vital signs during the procedure.

Routine care. After the procedure, your primary responsibilities include monitoring the patient for signs of an adverse reaction. Check his vital signs and notify the doctor immediately of any adverse reaction to the anesthetic or sedative.

Place the conscious patient in semi-Fowler's position; place the unconscious patient on his side, with the head of the bed slightly elevated to prevent aspiration, as ordered. Provide an emesis basin and instruct the patient to spit out saliva rather than swallow it. Observe sputum for blood, and notify the doctor immediately if excessive bleeding occurs.

Instruct the patient who has had a biopsy not to clear his throat or cough, because this may dislodge the clot at the biopsy site and cause hemorrhaging.

Restrict food and fluids until the gag reflex returns (usually in 2 hours). Then allow the patient to resume his usual diet, beginning with sips of clear liquid or ice chips.

Reassure the patient that postprocedural hoarseness, voice loss, or sore throat are temporary. Provide lozenges or a soothing liquid gargle to ease this discomfort when his gag reflex returns.

Performing emergency cricothyrotomy

In an emergency, you may be able to save a patient's life by establishing an airway through the cricothyroid membrane. To perform this emergency procedure, tilt the patient's chin up, and locate the cricothyroid membrane between the thyroid cartilage and the cricoid cartilage, as shown below. Carefully insert a scalpel or other sharp object through the skin and the cricothyroid membrane, into the trachea. Then insert a tube through the opening.

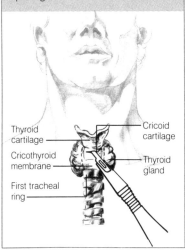

Thyroid cartilage
Cricothyroid membrane
First tracheal ring
Cricoid cartilage
Thyroid gland

Complications. Complications resulting from bronchoscopy include bleeding, infection, and pneumothorax.

Immediately report any subcutaneous crepitus around the patient's face and neck—a possible indication of tracheal or bronchial perforation. Also watch for and immediately report signs of respiratory difficulty, such as laryngeal stridor and dyspnea resulting from laryngeal edema or laryngospasm. Observe for signs

of hypoxemia (cyanosis), pneumothorax (dyspnea, cyanosis, diminished breath sounds on the affected side), and bronchospasm (hemoptysis).

Keep resuscitative equipment and a tracheotomy tray available for 24 hours after the procedure.

Cricothyrotomy

An emergency procedure, cricothyrotomy involves creating an opening in the trachea through the cricothyroid membrane. It's performed to gain rapid entry into the patient's airway for short-term ventilation until a definitive airway can be established.

To perform a cricothyrotomy, the doctor, a specially trained nurse, or other trained medical personnel will open the cricothyroid membrane with a scalpel or puncture it with an 11G needle or a special emergency tracheotomy needle. Ideally, it's done using sterile technique, but this may be impossible in an emergency outside the hospital.

Usually, you'll assist with the procedure. If no doctor is available, however, you may need to perform the cricothyrotomy yourself, provided that you're specially trained.

Indications. A cricothyrotomy is performed to establish an airway when special circumstances—such as laryngospasm or lack of equipment—prohibit endotracheal intubation or a conventional tracheotomy.

Performing cricothyrotomy. First obtain emergency equipment, including sterile gloves, povidone-iodine solution, sterile $4'' \times 4''$ gauze sponges, tape, a stethoscope, and a scalpel and Delabrode dilator, an 11G needle, or a tracheotomy needle. Then follow these steps:
• Put on the gloves. Then extend the

patient's head and neck to expose the incision site and provide proper tracheal position.

• Prepare the neck with a gauze sponge soaked in povidone-iodine solution. Then slide your thumb and fingers down the patient's neck to find his thyroid gland. You'll know you've located its outer borders when the space between your fingers and thumb widens. Move your index finger across the center of the gland, over the anterior edge of the cricoid ring.

• Make the incision into the cricothyroid membrane, just below the cricoid ring, and insert a Delabrode dilator to prevent tissues from closing around the incision. Or insert the 11G needle or tracheotomy needle into the cricothyroid membrane, and direct the needle downward and posteriorly to avoid damaging the vocal cords. Tape the dilator or needle in place.

• Auscultate bilaterally for breath sounds and take vital signs. (See *Performing emergency cricothyrotomy*.)

To perform an emergency cricothyrotomy outside the hospital, follow these steps:

• If you have gloves, put them on and locate the proper site, as described above.

• Cut or stab the patient's cricothyroid membrane using scissors or a pocket knife. Insert something hollow — for example, a drinking straw or plastic pen with ink cartridge removed — to keep the airway open.

• When you transfer the patient to an ambulance, give the attendant a verbal report.

• After you achieve ventilation and the patient gets to the hospital, a doctor or other trained medical personnel can insert another airway.

• Document the incident, including the date, time, events necessitating the procedure, and the patient's vital signs.

Routine care. Immediately after cricothyrotomy, watch for excessive bleeding at the insertion site, subcutaneous emphysema or inadequate ventilation from incorrect placement of equipment, and tracheal or vocal cord damage.

Complications. Infection may occur several days after this procedure, especially if sterile technique was compromised.

Suggested readings

Albarran-Sotelo, R., et al. *Textbook of Advanced Cardiac Life Support.* Dallas: American Heart Asociation, 1987.

Cardiopulmonary Emergencies. Springhouse, Pa.: Springhouse Corp., 1991.

Carroll, P.F. "Lowering the Risks of Endotracheal Suctioning," *Nursing88* 18(5):46-50, May 1988.

Goodnough, S.K. "Reducing Tracheal Injury and Aspiration," *DCCN* 7(6):324-32, November/December, 1988.

McHugh, J. "Perfecting the 3 Steps of Chest Physiotherapy," *Nursing87* 17(11):54-57, November 1987.

Miracle, V.A., and Allnut, D.R. "How to Perform Basic Airway Management," *Nursing90* 20(4):55-60, April 1990.

4

OXYGEN DELIVERY

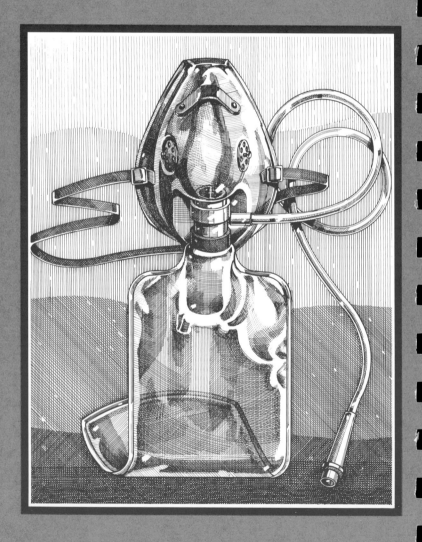

Today, many hospital patients require supplemental oxygen therapy — delivery of oxygen at a concentration above the 21% present in room air. Patients may receive this therapy for any of these reasons:

• to ensure sufficient oxygen to meet metabolic needs at the cellular level, particularly when oxygen demands increase, as in fever or massive tissue repair

• to correct hypoxemia by making increased alveolar oxygen available for diffusion when disorders such as atelectasis or adult respiratory distress syndrome impair diffusion

• to decrease the work of breathing necessary to maintain adequate oxygenation by correcting hypoxemia

• to diminish the myocardial work load by correcting hypoxemia, especially when myocardial tissues are already compromised — such as after a myocardial infarction or during cardiac arrhythmias

• to improve oxygenation in patients with decreased blood oxygen-carrying capacity, such as occurs in anemia, carbon monoxide poisoning, or sickle cell disease.

Like most drugs, oxygen requires a doctor's order and carries some potentially serious hazards. For instance, an oxygen overdose can be as dangerous as any drug overdose — especially in vulnerable patients, such as those with chronic obstructive pulmonary disease (COPD). Thus, safe, effective oxygen therapy hinges largely on your knowledge of oxygen delivery systems and respiratory care.

This chapter covers the basics of oxygen therapy, including oxygen delivery systems, humidifiers and nebulizers, and special devices for pediatric patients. It also explains how to set up the equipment, administer oxygen, troubleshoot problems, and manage complications.

Oxygen delivery systems

These systems come in two basic types: low-flow and high-flow. *Low-flow systems* provide oxygen to supplement the oxygen the patient receives from room air. They include nasal cannulas, simple face masks, and rebreather masks. *High-flow systems*, such as the Venturi mask, provide all the oxygen necessary to meet the patient's inspiratory requirements.

Other oxygen delivery systems — including the trach collar or mask, face tent, transtracheal catheter, and T tube — provide high humidification as well as high oxygen flow. Specially designed oxygen delivery devices meet the specific needs of neonates and children. These special delivery systems — Isolettes, oxygen hoods, and croup tents — completely envelop the child in a high-oxygen environment, ensuring compliance with supplemental oxygen therapy.

Each oxygen delivery system has particular indications, advantages, and disadvantages and delivers a specific percentage of oxygen. (See *Comparing oxygen delivery systems,* pages 108 and 109.) Safe, effective therapy hinges on the proper choice of delivery system and oxygen concentration for the patient's condition.

You should also be aware that oxygen delivery systems are increasingly being used in the home setting. This has resulted from changes in insurance reimbursement and shortened hospital stays. Home

(Text continues on page 110.)

Comparing oxygen delivery systems

Several types of oxygen delivery systems are available, each with its own benefits, drawbacks, and indications for use. The following chart compares the advantages and disadvantages of these systems.

TYPE	ADVANTAGES	DISADVANTAGES
Nasal cannula	• Safe and simple • Comfortable; easily tolerated • Nasal prongs can be shaped to fit facial contour. • Effective for delivering low oxygen concentrations • Allows freedom of movement; doesn't interfere with eating or talking • Inexpensive; disposable • Can provide continuous positive airway pressure (CPAP) for infants and children	• Can't deliver oxygen concentrations greater than 40% • Can't be used when patient has complete nasal obstruction; for example, mucosal edema or polyps • May cause headaches or dry mucous membranes if flow rate exceeds 6 liters/minute • Can dislodge easily • Strap may pinch patient's chin if adjusted too tightly. • Patient must be alert and cooperative to help keep cannula in place.
Simple face mask	• Can deliver oxygen concentration of 40% to 60%	• Hot and confining; may irritate the patient's skin • Tight seal required for higher oxygen concentration may cause discomfort. • Interferes with eating and talking • Impractical for long-term therapy because of imprecision
Partial rebreather mask	• Openings in mask allow patient to inhale room air if oxygen source fails. • Effectively delivers high oxygen concentrations (35% to 60%)	• Tight seal required for accurate oxygen concentration may cause discomfort. • Interferes with eating and talking • Hot and confining; may irritate the patient's skin • Bag may twist or kink. • Impractical for long-term therapy
Nonrebreather mask	• Delivers the highest possible oxygen concentration (60% to 90%) short of intubation and mechanical ventilation • Effective for short-term therapy • Doesn't dry mucous membranes • Can be converted to a partial rebreather mask, if necessary, by removing one-way flap	• Requires a tight seal, which may be difficult to maintain and may cause discomfort • May irritate the patient's skin • Impractical for long-term therapy

Comparing oxygen delivery systems *(continued)*

TYPE	ADVANTAGES	DISADVANTAGES
Venturi mask	• Delivers highly accurate oxygen concentrations despite patient's respiratory pattern because the same amount of air is always entrained • Diluter jets can be changed or dial turned to change oxygen concentration • Doesn't dry mucous membranes • Humidity or aerosol can be added to the Venturi stream.	• Confining and may irritate skin • Oxygen concentration may be altered if mask doesn't fit snugly, if tubing kinks, if oxygen intake ports become blocked, if less-than-recommended liter flow is used, or if patient is hyperpneic. • Interferes with eating and talking • Condensate may collect and drain on patient if humidification is being used.
CPAP mask	• Noninvasively improves arterial oxygenation by increasing functional residual capacity • Provides continuous positive airway pressure in the nonintubated patient • Patient can talk and cough without interrupting positive pressure.	• Mask feels uncomfortable and confining. • Continuous positive airway pressure may be lost if mask doesn't fit snugly. • Heightened risk of aspiration if patient vomits • Increased risk of pneumothorax, diminished cardiac output, and gastric distention • May worsen patient anxiety
Trach collar or mask	• Can be used to administer high humidity • Swivel adapter allows tubing to attach on either side. • Frontal port permits suctioning. • Elastic ties allow you to pull mask from tracheostomy without removing it. • Gas can be heated or cooled.	• Any condensate collected may drain into tracheostomy. • Secretions collected in the collar may result in an infected stoma.
Face tent	• Administers high humidity • Functions as high-flow system when attached to a Venturi nebulizer • Substitutes for face mask if patient can't tolerate a covered nose – for example, because of a broken nose or facial burns • Doesn't dry mucous membranes • Gas can be heated or cooled.	• May irritate skin • Interferes with eating and talking • Doesn't deliver precise oxygen concentrations without Venturi attachment; patient can rebreathe carbon dioxide unless a Venturi system is used. • Impractical for long-term therapy
T tube	• Offers high humidity when connected to a nebulizer • Allows greater patient mobility • Can be used for tracheostomy or endotracheal tube • Functions as a high-flow system when attached to a Venturi system • Gas can be heated or cooled.	• May stick to tracheostomy (from humidity or secretions) • Any condensate collected in the tube may drain into tracheostomy. • Weight of T tube can pull on the tracheostomy tube.

Guide to home oxygen therapy

Before discharging a patient who will receive home oxygen therapy, make sure you know the types of oxygen therapy, the kinds of services that are available to him, and the service schedules offered by local home suppliers.

If your patient will be discharged with oxygen for the first time, make sure his health insurance covers home oxygen. If it doesn't, find out what criteria he must meet to obtain coverage. Without a third-party payment, home oxygen therapy may be prohibitively expensive.

Home oxygen therapy can be given using an oxygen tank, an oxygen concentrator, or liquid oxygen.

Oxygen tank

Commonly used for patients who need oxygen on a standby basis or who need a ventilator at home, the oxygen tank has several disadvantages, including its cumbersome design and the need for frequent refills. Because oxygen is stored under high pressure, the oxygen tank also poses a potential hazard.

Oxygen concentrator

The oxygen concentrator operates electrically and extracts oxygen molecules from room air. It can be used for low oxygen flow (less than 4 liters/minute) and doesn't need to be refilled with oxygen. However, the oxygen concentrator won't work during a power failure.

Liquid oxygen

This option is commonly used by patients who are oxygen-dependent but still mobile. The system includes a large liquid reservoir for home use. When the patient wants to leave the house, he fills a portable unit worn over the shoulder; this supplies oxygen for up to several hours, depending on the liter flow.

oxygen therapy requires good communication among the health care providers who will develop a plan of care for the patient. (See *Guide to home oxygen therapy*.)

Basic concerns

Although oxygen delivery systems differ somewhat in design and operation, initial equipment setup and basic nursing care are similar for all systems. Typically, each hospital has a different type of oxygen access and oxygen therapy equipment, so be sure to check your hospital's policy and the equipment manufacturer's directions for specific instructions.

Setting up. First, assess the patient's respiratory status to determine the need for oxygen therapy and to establish a baseline for subsequent assessments. Then obtain the appropriate equipment. If you're unfamiliar with the equipment, contact the respiratory therapy department or appropriate personnel for assistance.

Ensure a safe environment for oxygen administration—no open flames or potential sources of sparks. Post oxygen precaution signs over the patient's bed and outside the room, and explain the precautions to the patient and all other persons who will enter the room. Remember that while oxygen itself isn't flammable, it will feed a fire.

Be sure to explain the procedure to the patient. Remember, he'll probably be anxious because of his breathing difficulty. Placing a mask over his nose and mouth may exacerbate this anxiety.

In most cases, you'll follow these basic steps when setting up oxygen equipment:

• Wash your hands before (and

Preparing and maintaining oxygen cylinders

If your hospital doesn't have wall units, you'll probably use a cylinder to deliver oxygen. Here's how you set up and use a cylinder.

Setting up

• Check the cylinder gauge to ensure an adequate oxygen supply. When the cylinder is full, the gauge should read 2,200 psi.

• Remove the valve cover. With the oxygen spout pointing away from you, "crack" the cylinder by opening the valve slightly to blow any dust from the spout lip; then immediately shut the valve.

• Connect the pressure-reduction gauge to equalize pressure between the tank and the flowmeter, and attach the flowmeter if the pressure gauge lacks one. Then turn the gauge's flow-control knob counter-clockwise to open it, and slowly open the valve on top of the cylinder until the pressure gauge needle stops moving.

• Next, turn the flow-control knob clockwise until the flowmeter dial shows the prescribed flow rate in liters/minute. Then turn the flow-control knob counter-clockwise until the flowmeter needle falls to zero.

• Transport the cylinder to the bedside in a cylinder cart. Keep the cylinder secured and away from heat to prevent it from breaking or exploding.

• If using a humidifier, fill the humidifier bottle two-thirds full with sterile distilled water. Screw the filled humidifier bottle to its adapter and connect it to the flowmeter. Turn on the oxygen to 2 or 3 liters/minute and watch for bubbles in the distilled water to ensure humidifier patency.

Nursing considerations

• During oxygen therapy, change the humidifier bottle setup and sterile distilled water according to hospital policy. Replace the water in a reusable bottle to prevent bacterial growth. Discard and replace a commercially prepared bottle. Make sure the patient is comfortable; some humidification systems produce a strong chill.

• Always calculate the length of time that the cylinder will supply oxygen. If necessary, have a second cylinder available for a quick switch when the first runs out.

• Warn the patient and all other persons in the room not to smoke or use an improperly grounded radio, TV, or electric razor. If using the cylinder at home, make sure all electrical equipment is inspected and properly grounded.

after) initiating oxygen therapy to guard against transmitting nosocomial infection.

• When using a wall unit, connect the adapter to the unit and check for leaks; reinsert, if necessary. Attach the flowmeter and turn on the control switch to ensure that the flowmeter is working, then shut it off again.

• If you're using an oxygen cylinder, turn on the cylinder. (See *Preparing and maintaining oxygen cylinders*

for more information.)

• If you're providing humidification, fill the humidifier bottle or reservoir two-thirds full with sterile distilled water. (Avoid tap water and saline solution, which will leave mineral deposits in the equipment.) Fill only to the marker — overfilling will cause water to flow back into the oxygen gauges. If you're using a prefilled bottle, check that the seal is unbroken; then listen for the rushing sound of the released vacuum as you unseal the bottle. If you don't hear this sound, discard the bottle—it may not be sterile. Screw the filled humidifier bottle to its adapter.

• Connect the humidifier bottle to the tubing and the flowmeter. Set the flowmeter as ordered, making sure the center of the ball is on the line indicating the prescribed liters per minute. Be careful not to exceed the safe limit of 6 liters/minute. Humidification may not be used in very low-flow oxygen therapy (1 to 2 liters/minute); ambient humidification may be adequate.

• Now begin giving oxygen, following your hospital's protocols and the equipment manufacturer's instructions.

• Document all your actions and the patient's responses. Compare ongoing assessment findings to the patient's baseline data.

• After discontinuing oxygen, discard disposable equipment according to hospital guidelines, and send any reusable equipment to the proper department for sterilization.

Nursing care. For all patients receiving supplemental oxygen, perform a respiratory assessment—including monitoring arterial blood gas (ABG) levels and arterial oxygen saturation (SaO_2), if appropriate—at least every 8 hours to determine the effectiveness of treatment. If the patient has a history of respiratory disorders, such as asthma, COPD, or pneumonia, or a history of congestive heart failure, assess him every 4 hours. If you detect a problem, or if his condition worsens, notify the doctor and monitor the patient more closely.

Be sure to refer to your hospital's policy for taking the temperature of a patient receiving oxygen. Studies show that only a small decline

in body temperature occurs during oxygen administration. Given this small change and the discomfort caused by rectal thermometers, many clinicians believe that taking rectal temperatures isn't warranted. Because of this small drop in temperature, many clinicians also believe that oxygen therapy shouldn't be discontinued when taking oral temperatures. Of course, if your patient can't hold an oral thermometer in the proper position, or if you question the accuracy of the temperature, rectal temperature measurement may be necessary.

Complications. When caring for a patient receiving oxygen therapy, monitor him for the following complications.

• *Respiratory depression.* In a patient with COPD, hypoxia provides the main stimulus for breathing. Too much oxygen can remove that stimulus, leading to apnea. Avoid giving high concentrations of oxygen, and provide only enough fraction of inspired oxygen (FIO_2) to maintain the patient's partial pressure of oxygen in arterial blood (PaO_2) in a safe range. Monitor for somnolence, diminished respiratory rate, and other signs of impending respiratory depression, and keep emergency resuscitation equipment available.

• *Circulatory depression.* In a patient with COPD, hypoxia can produce generalized vasoconstriction. Oxygen therapy reverses this condition and dilates the blood vessels, possibly causing a significant decline in blood pressure. During oxygen therapy, closely monitor the patient's blood pressure and cardiovascular status, and instruct him to change positions slowly to help prevent injury stemming from the effects of orthostatic hypotension.

• *Absorption atelectasis.* Administering very high oxygen concentrations will wash nitrogen from the patient's lungs during oxygen exchange, possibly leading to absorption atelectasis. Help prevent this problem by having the patient deep-breathe frequently; this hyperinflates the lungs and helps prevent alveolar collapse.

• *Oxygen toxicity.* When a patient receives a high concentration of oxygen for a prolonged period, serious lung damage (and, in neonates, blindness) can occur. To prevent this, intervene to improve the patient's ventilation with chest physiotherapy and suctioning. Monitor ABG values and PaO_2 to ensure optimal oxygenation with the least amount of oxygen delivered.

• *Hypoxia.* When discontinuing treatment, monitor the patient for signs of hypoxia, such as tachycardia, confusion, restlessness, headache, and lethargy, which may indicate the need to reinstitute oxygen therapy.

Nasal cannula

The most frequently used oxygen delivery system, the nasal cannula delivers low-flow oxygen through two plastic prongs that fit into the patient's nostrils. (See *Nasal cannula.*) To use a nasal cannula, the patient must be breathing spontaneously with a normal tidal volume and have no airway obstruction that could interfere with gas delivery to the lungs.

Comfortable, unobtrusive, and relatively inexpensive, the nasal cannula delivers between 24% and 44% oxygen concentration.

A patient receiving supplemental oxygen via nasal cannula is susceptible to several complications, including mucous membrane dryness and skin or sinus irritation from the delivery device.

Nasal cannula

Simple, inexpensive, and easy to use, the nasal cannula allows the patient to talk, eat, and drink. It consists of tubing, nasal prongs and, on some devices, an elastic strap.

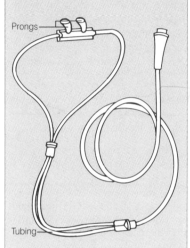

Setting up. To start therapy with a nasal cannula, follow these steps:

• Inspect each nostril using a flashlight. Check for patency, polyps, edema, and deviated septum or other obstruction. If both nostrils are obstructed, you'll need to deliver the oxygen via a mask.

• Check whether the nasal prongs are straight, smooth, or curved. Also check whether one side is smoother or flatter than the other. If the prongs are straight, and if both sides are the same, place them in the patient's nostrils with either side up. If they're straight, but the sides are different, place the smoother or flatter side against the patient's skin because it will produce less friction. Place curved prongs with the curve facing toward the nostrils' floor. This position helps prevent obstruction of the cannula lumen by the nasal mucosa, which can decrease oxygen flow.

• Now hook the cannula tubing behind the patient's ears and under his chin. Then slide the adjuster upward to hold the cannula in place. When using an elastic strap to hold the cannula in place, position the strap over the patient's head above his ears. With either method, avoid securing the cannula too tightly; this can lead to pressure sores or occlusion of the nasal prongs.

Nursing care. At least every 8 hours or whenever it becomes soiled, remove the cannula and wipe it with a wet cloth. While doing so, inspect the prongs for patency.

As with any oxygen delivery system, be sure to monitor the nasal cannula tubing for kinking or occlusion. Most nasal tubing humidification systems have a safety pressure release valve. If for any reason the oxygen tubing becomes pinched or occluded — such as from the patient sitting on the tubing or the tubing catching in the bed's side rails — backward positive pressure flows into the humidification bottle and out the positive pressure release valve. This flow creates a high-pitched "whistling" sound alerting you to an obstructed oxygen line.

Transtracheal catheter

In transtracheal oxygen therapy, a catheter is inserted into an opening at the base of the patient's neck and held in place with a thin chain necklace that runs through two openings in the catheter flange. When connected to an oxygen source, the catheter delivers oxygen directly into the trachea. Because the catheter can be concealed by a

shirt or scarf, it's often preferred by patients requiring long-term oxygen therapy. Also, because oxygen enters the trachea directly, reducing the amount that escapes into the atmosphere, this system conserves oxygen and can reduce monthly therapy costs.

Transtracheal oxygen therapy usually is indicated for the same patients who might otherwise receive continuous nasal cannula therapy or face mask oxygen at home. In particular, it benefits patients who require improved mobility; resist or won't comply with nasal cannula therapy; prefer the comfort, convenience, and appearance of a concealed catheter; or experience complications from nasal cannula therapy.

Insertion. In most cases, transtracheal catheter insertion can be performed on an outpatient basis. Using local anesthesia, the doctor makes a small incision and inserts a needle into the trachea. After aspirating air to confirm needle placement in the trachea, the doctor inserts a guide wire through the needle, removes the needle, dilates the new opening (called a transtracheal tract), and inserts a thin plastic stent over the guide wire. (See *Transtracheal catheter.*) The stent keeps the tract patent during the initial healing period but does not deliver oxygen. Finally, the doctor removes the wire and sutures the stent in place. A neck X-ray confirms catheter placement.

After 1 week, the doctor removes the stent and inserts a scoop 1 catheter into the tract. A #9 French catheter with a single port at the tip, the scoop 1 can be cleaned in place while the tract matures, which usually takes 6 to 8 weeks. After this time, the patient may elect to continue using the scoop 1 catheter if cleaning in place is desirable; if not, the doctor will insert a scoop 2 catheter.

Designed for use in a mature tract when removal for cleaning is both feasible and desirable, the scoop 2 is a #8 French catheter with a single end port and six side ports. These ports deliver oxygen in a "shower" effect above the carina, distributing oxygen more evenly than a scoop 1—an advantage at resting flow rates above 6 liters/minute.

Nursing care. Your care of a transtracheal catheter includes evaluating ABG levels and teaching your patient about therapy.
• *Evaluating blood gases.* Before starting transtracheal oxygen therapy, obtain ABG values or a pulse oximetry reading to titrate the oxygen flow rate and determine whether the patient is hypoxic or retaining carbon dioxide (CO_2). In most patients, SaO_2 should be between 91% and 95% and PaO_2 between 65 and 80 mm Hg, both at rest and after exercise.
• *Patient teaching.* During transtracheal oxygen therapy, you'll teach the patient how to use and care for his transtracheal oxygen catheter.

Explain how he'll care for the tract opening by cleaning it daily with a cotton-tipped swab dipped in hydrogen peroxide. Tell him to use a mild soap to wash his neck, even after the tract matures. (Like a tracheostomy, a transtracheal tract never totally heals as long as it's kept open for oxygen delivery.)

Be sure to tell the patient that scoop catheters must be replaced every 2 to 3 months because they become brittle after prolonged use. Discuss how to keep the transtra-

EQUIPMENT

Transtracheal catheter

The transtracheal catheter has three components: the stent, the scoop 1, and the scoop 2.

Stent	Scoop 1	Scoop 2

cheal catheter patent and how to recognize complications and intervene if they occur.

Complications. During transtracheal oxygen therapy, monitor the patient for the following complications.
• *Catheter obstruction.* Observe for unusual shortness of breath, coughing, or dyspnea, which may indicate that the catheter is obstructed or

pointing upward in the trachea. Difficulty irrigating the catheter, a whistling sound from the oxygen tank's humidifier, or a sudden escape of oxygen when disconnecting the catheter from the oxygen tubes could indicate obstruction. Instruct the patient to promptly report any such problems.

• *Infection.* Monitor for signs and symptoms of infection, such as fever, redness and swelling in the tract opening, and purulent drainage. Expect to administer an antibiotic agent to treat infection.

• *Bronchospasm.* Observe for increased wheezing and shortness of breath. Bronchodilator drugs may be prescribed if needed to treat wheezing. Again, the catheter should be checked for obstruction if these symptoms occur.

• *Subcutaneous emphysema.* This complication may develop if oxygen moves backward and upward into the tissue lining the neck. A layer of epithelial tissue forms within a few weeks, lining the tract and preventing this complication. Withholding transtracheal oxygen delivery until 1 week after the insertion procedure will reduce the risk of subcutaneous emphysema.

• *Decannulation.* Placing small strips of tape over the chain on either side of the catheter for the first couple of weeks after the procedure can decrease the risk of decannulation.

Cleaning the catheter. Because the scoop 2 must be removed twice a day for cleaning, it can't be used until the transtracheal tract matures. Some patients prefer to continue using the scoop 1 because it requires cleaning only once a week.

To clean a *scoop 1 catheter*, follow these steps:

• First, wash your hands to help prevent transmission of nosocomial infection, then place a nasal cannula on the patient to provide oxygen during the procedure. Disconnect the oxygen tubing from the catheter and connect it to the nasal cannula.

• Next, irrigate the catheter with 1.5 ml of normal saline solution. Insert a cleaning rod previously washed with antimicrobial soap into the catheter and advance it as far as possible. Then pull it back. Repeat this three times.

• Remove the rod, then instill 1.5 ml of normal saline solution into the catheter. Reconnect the oxygen tubing to the catheter.

• Finally, clean the rod with antimicrobial soap and store it in a dry place.

To clean a *scoop 2 catheter*, follow these steps:

• After washing your hands, discontinue the oxygen and administer oxygen via a nasal cannula, as with the scoop 1 catheter.

• Lubricate a second scoop 2 catheter with water-soluble jelly. Remove the existing scoop 2 catheter and immediately replace it with the second one. Secure the newly inserted catheter on the necklace and reinstitute the oxygen.

• Clean the catheter you just removed in antimicrobial soap under tepid tap water. Air dry, then store it in a dry place.

Oxygen masks

When not under positive pressure, oxygen masks can deliver up to 90% oxygen and are indicated for patients with nasal obstructions and for those who require high amounts of FIO_2 or humidification. The cone-shaped oxygen mask fits snugly over the patient's mouth and nose with an adjustable strap. Most patients find the masks confining and a hindrance to eating and talking. These disadvantages may reduce patient compliance, decreasing the percentage of oxygen delivered.

Mask selection. Oxygen masks come in four basic types: the simple face mask, the nonrebreather mask, the partial rebreather mask, and the Venturi mask (see *Types of oxygen masks*, pages 118 and 119).

• *Simple face mask.* Equipped with an oxygen entry port and multiple exhalation ports, the simple face mask can deliver only moderate percentages of oxygen (40% to 60%). It's indicated for patients unable to use a nasal cannula, such as those with a nasal obstruction or those who are mouth-breathing.

• *Nonrebreather and partial rebreather masks.* Used for patients requiring a high percentage of oxygen, the nonrebreather mask and the partial rebreather mask deliver high oxygen concentrations using slightly different principles.

The nonrebreather mask delivers up to 90% oxygen — the highest possible oxygen concentration short of positive pressure ventilation or intubation with mechanical ventilation. It also can be used to administer other gas mixtures, such as CO_2 and helium.

This device contains three one-way flaps: one located between the reservoir bag and the mask and two others on the mask itself. Oxygen flows from the source into the bag. Then, when the patient inhales, the flap between the bag and mask lifts up, allowing the patient to inspire the oxygen from the bag. Simultaneously, the flaps on the mask close, preventing inspiration of room air. When the patient exhales, the bag flap closes, preventing CO_2 from entering the reservoir bag, and the flaps on the mask open to release expired air to the atmosphere.

In contrast, the partial rebreather mask doesn't have the nonrebreather's one-way flaps on the mask or the bag. So this mask conserves roughly the first third of the patient's exhaled air, which flows into the reservoir bag. Along with oxygen, the patient also rebreathes his exhaled air, which — because it comes from the trachea and bronchi and does not participate in gas exchange in the lungs — is high in oxygen concentration. This allows the partial rebreather mask to deliver up to 60% oxygen.

• *Venturi mask.* Delivering a precise oxygen concentration to within 1%, the Venturi mask is especially useful in administering oxygen to patients with COPD. With this device, oxygen enters the tubing at a prescribed flow rate. When oxygen reaches the Venturi device, it meets a restricted orifice. To maintain the same flow rate, the velocity increases, decreasing pressure on the tubing walls and allowing room air to be drawn in from the ports of entrainment on the side of the Venturi device. The amount of air entrained depends on the size of the orifice. The smaller the orifice, the larger the increase in velocity, the larger the decrease in pressure, and the larger the amount of room air entrained — and, consequently, the greater the oxygen dilution and the lower the FIO_2.

Setting up. To set up an oxygen mask, first select the size mask that offers the most comfortable fit and best airtight seal for your patient. Then follow these steps:

• Connect the tubing, mask, and humidification device to the flowmeter (unless using a Venturi mask, which usually doesn't require hu-

Types of oxygen masks

Illustrated below are the four basic types of oxygen masks you may use.

Simple face mask
This inexpensive and relatively comfortable device delivers moderate oxygen concentrations.

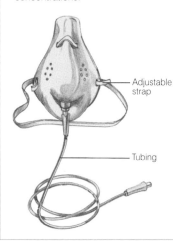

Adjustable strap

Tubing

Nonrebreather mask
This mask, which can deliver up to 90% oxygen, has three one-way flaps: one located between the mask and the reservoir bag, the other two on the mask itself.

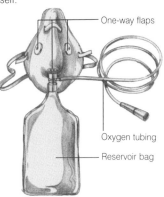

One-way flaps

Oxygen tubing

Reservoir bag

midification). Set the flowmeter to the correct setting to deliver the prescribed oxygen concentration. (Remember, the flow rate must be at least 5 liters/minute to adequately flush CO_2 from the mask.)
• Place the mask over the patient's mouth, nose, and chin. Press the flexible nosepiece down over the bridge of the nose to provide a tight seal, then adjust the elastic band over the head above the ears so the mask fits snugly on the face. To ensure a tight seal, plug any gaps with gauze pads. Without a tight seal, room air may enter on inspiration and dilute the percentage of FIO_2 delivered.
• For a *simple face mask,* set the flowmeter to supply the prescribed

oxygen rate. Unlike some of the other masks, a simple face mask requires a doctor's order specifying the oxygen flow rate to be administered.
• For a *nonrebreather or partial rebreather mask,* set the flowmeter to the ordered setting, usually between 6 and 15 liters/minute, depending on the oxygen concentration the patient requires. (See *Determining oxygen percentages by liter flow,* page 120.)

Observe the reservoir bag for initial inflation. If using a nonrebreather mask, ensure that the one-way flaps operate properly. Refer to your hospital's policy for setting up a nonrebreather mask. Some hospitals require the removal of one

Partial rebreather mask

The partial rebreather mask, which can deliver up to 60% oxygen, has no one-way flaps on the bag or mask. It's designed to conserve roughly the first third of a patient's exhaled air, which flows into the reservoir bag.

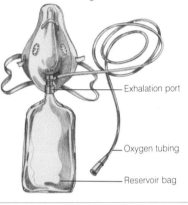

Exhalation port

Oxygen tubing

Reservoir bag

Venturi mask

The Venturi mask uses a jet adapter and entrainment collector to deliver precise oxygen concentrations at high flow rates.

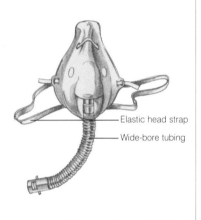

Elastic head strap

Wide-bore tubing

flap as a safety measure; that way, if the oxygen source becomes discontinued, the patient can still inspire room air.

As the patient breathes, observe the reservoir bag; it should deflate slightly on inspiration.

• For a *Venturi mask,* select the correct jet adapter for the percentage of FIO_2 ordered, or dial in the percentage ordered. Connect the tubing from the oxygen source to the Venturi adapter, then set the appropriate liter flow following the specific mask guidelines.

If humidification has been ordered for the patient, connect the wide-bore tubing to the jet adapter and the humidification device to the flowmeter before hooking up the oxygen source.

Nursing care. To help increase compliance with oxygen therapy, explain the purpose of the mask to the patient and make him as comfortable as possible. During oxygen delivery, frequently check that the mask is properly positioned and airtight. Adjust it as needed.

When using a nonrebreather mask, watch the flaps for movement; the reservoir bag flap should rise on inspiration and close on expiration, whereas the mask flaps should close on inspiration and rise on expiration. Also observe the reservoir bag to ensure that it's full and deflates only slightly as the patient breathes.

Determining oxygen percentages by liter flow

To determine the approximate oxygen concentration that can be administered via each delivery device, line up the oxygen delivery rate, given as liters per minute, with the delivery method. Remember, these figures apply only to patients breathing at a normal rate and rhythm and at a tidal volume of about 500 ml. An X indicates that a rate can't be reached with a particular delivery method.

		DELIVERY METHOD					
		Nasal cannula/ catheter	Simple mask	Partial rebreather mask	Non- rebreather mask	Croup tent	Isolette (standard use)
OXYGEN DELIVERY RATE (liters/minute)	2	23% to 28%	X	X	X	X	X
	3	28% to 30%	X	X	X	X	X
	4	32% to 36%	X	X	X	X	X
	5	40%	40%	X	X	X	X
	6	Maxi- mum of 44%	45% to 50%	35%	55% to 60%	X	35% to 40% (with flag up); 80% to 90% (with flag down)
	8	X	55% to 60%	45% to 50%	60% to 80%	X	40% (with flag up); 95% to 100% (with flag down)
	10	X	X	60%	80% to 90%	30% to 40%	40% (with flag up); 95% to 100% (with flag down)
	12	X	X	60%	90%	40% to 50%	X
	15	X	X	60%	90%	50%	X

If the reservoir bag deflates markedly on inspiration, increase the oxygen flow rate slightly. If the bag continues to deflate, check all connections to ensure unimpeded oxygen flow into the reservoir bag.

When using any mask with a reservoir bag, take care to prevent the bag from twisting or kinking. Make sure that the bag is visible and can expand freely. Avoid using high humidification on a mask with a reservoir bag unless an in-line water bag is available. If water collects in the in-line bag or the reservoir bag, empty it. Remove the connecting tubing from the humidification device, drain the tubing into a graduate cylinder or other container, and properly dispose of the fluid.

With a Venturi mask, periodically check the Venturi adapter for the proper setting. Prevent kinks in the tubing and keep the entrainment port from being covered by the patient's gown or a blanket.

If you suspect an improperly functioning Venturi device, check all connections for tightness. Make sure that the entrainment port isn't blocked and, if using humidification, check the tubing for condensation, which can cause plugging.

Before removing the oxygen mask so the patient can eat, ask the doctor to order a nasal cannula for use during meals. After discontinuing oxygen delivery via mask, be prepared to continue delivery using some other device — in most cases, a nasal cannula.

Complications. Besides monitoring for complications of oxygen therapy, also assess for these complications specific to mask use.

• *Skin irritation and pressure sores.* Remove the mask frequently and inspect the skin for irritation and breakdown. Wipe the mask with a wet cloth and clean the patient's face.

If necessary, apply gauze pads to the mask edges to decrease skin irritation, and cut away part of the upper mask to keep it away from the patient's eyes. (Be sure to check

the manufacturer's guidelines before cutting the mask.)

When replacing the mask, be careful not to overtighten it.

• *Aspiration.* A patient using an oxygen mask — particularly an unconscious or semiconscious patient — is at increased risk for aspiration. If unable to remove the mask after vomiting, he could aspirate the vomitus contained in the mask on the next inspiration. Monitor an at-risk patient closely during oxygen therapy.

CPAP mask

As its name suggests, the continuous positive airway pressure (CPAP) mask provides positive pressure in the airways throughout the entire respiratory cycle. In a CPAP mask setup, flow comes from an air or oxygen source to the patient. (See *CPAP mask,* page 122.) He then exhales against resistance — which produces the positive pressure and creates back pressure in the lungs. The CPAP mask is indicated for a spontaneously breathing patient with severe hypoxemia caused by acute respiratory failure, atelectasis, pulmonary contusion, or sleep apnea.

Setting up. First, obtain the proper size mask with softsealing outer edges to fit snugly over the patient's face. Then follow these steps:
• Attach the flow generator to the oxygen outlet, then attach the air entrainment port to the flow generator and set the dial to the desired pressure. Next, attach the humidification system to the flow generator and tubing.
• Turn on the generator and adjust the FIO_2 dial to provide the desired flow; if necessary, use an oxygen analyzer to determine the correct setting.

CPAP mask

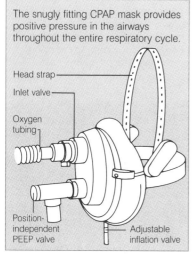

The snugly fitting CPAP mask provides positive pressure in the airways throughout the entire respiratory cycle.

Head strap

Inlet valve

Oxygen tubing

Position-independent PEEP valve

Adjustable inflation valve

• Attach the oxygen tubing to the mask's inlet valve.
• If ordered, attach a positive end-expiratory pressure (PEEP) valve and dial in the ordered amount of PEEP.
• Finally, apply the mask, positioning one strap behind the patient's neck and the other strap over the head above the ears; ensure a snug but not overly tight fit.

Nursing care. During CPAP therapy, check the mask regularly to ensure a tight seal between the mask edges and the patient's skin. Because the tight seal required can lead to skin breakdown under the mask edges, be sure to remove the mask and inspect the skin periodically.

Many patients find the CPAP mask uncomfortable, confining, and a source of anxiety. Provide frequent reassurance and simple explanations of procedures to help reduce anxiety. Keep in mind that a hypoxemic patient may be confused as well as anxious.

If you note a decrease in positive pressure (the most common problem associated with the CPAP mask), check all equipment connections for tightness and ensure that the mask fits the patient snugly. If you can't obtain a good seal between the mask and the patient's skin, try another size mask. If you continue to have difficulty with the equipment, consult the respiratory care department or other appropriate personnel.

Complications. The high pressures delivered with the CPAP mask put the patient at risk for the following complications.
• *Gastric distention.* Air pushed into the stomach by positive pressure may cause gastric distention, which can increase the risk of stress ulcers in the already compromised patient. Assess the patient for signs of distention; he may need gastric decompression.
• *Decreased cardiac output.* Increased intrathoracic pressure produced by CPAP decreases venous return to the heart, causing a drop in blood pressure and cardiac output. Carefully monitor the patient's blood pressure and heart rate. If pressure drops more than 10 mm Hg, position the patient with his head below the level of his heart; if the pressure continues to drop, alert the doctor.
• *Tension pneumothorax.* During CPAP therapy, pneumothorax can occur as a result of the increased positive pressure on the lung tissue. Monitor for asymmetrical chest expansion, absent breath sounds on the affected side, tracheal deviation away from the affected side, hypoxia, cyanosis, tachycardia, tachy-

pnea, and distended neck veins. If you detect these signs, notify the doctor immediately and prepare to assist with chest tube insertion.
• *Hypoventilation.* In CPAP, the positive pressure causes overdistention of normal lung tissue and increases the ratio of dead space, possibly leading to CO_2 retention. To detect hypoventilation, monitor ABG values.

Trach collar
Sometimes called a trach mask, this device fits over a tracheostomy tube and delivers humidification and oxygen to a patient with a tracheostomy or laryngectomy who doesn't require mechanical ventilation.
The trach collar consists of a flexible collar-shaped device with an adjustable neck strap, a large-bore tubing connection, and a large exhalation port. (See *Trach collar.*) The device is designed to swivel so that the patient can move freely with it in place.

Setting up. To set up the trach collar, follow these steps:
• Attach the trach collar and tubing to the humidification device. If you'll be delivering heated humidity, turn on the heating device following the equipment manufacturer's instructions.
• Set the flowmeter at 10 liters/ minute.
• Slip the strap around the patient's neck and adjust the elastic ties so that the collar fits snugly over the tracheostomy tube.
• During oxygen delivery, readjust the flow rate as necessary to provide a visible mist.

Nursing care. This system's high humidification may produce significant condensation in the tubing. Empty the condensate frequently so

Trach collar

Designed to deliver humidified oxygen or air to a patient with a tracheostomy, the trach collar fits over the trach tube.

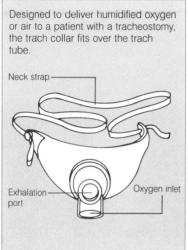

it cannot drain into the patient's tracheostomy, harbor and grow potentially dangerous organisms, or obstruct dependent sections of the tubing. To drain condensate, disconnect the tubing from the trach collar or the humidification device, drain the condensate into a container, and dispose of it properly. Never drain the condensate into the humidification system or the tracheostomy.
   If delivering heated humidity, monitor the mist temperature. Overheated aerosol can cause tracheal or pulmonary irritation or burns.

Face tent
A specialized type of face mask, the face tent provides oxygen and humidification for patients without artificial airways who can't tolerate pressure on the nose or face. (See *Face tent,* page 124.) This device has important advantages for some

Face tent

A shieldlike mask that fits loosely over the nose and mouth, the face tent provides humidified oxygen to patients who can't tolerate pressure on the nose or face.

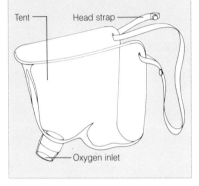

patients — such as those with a broken or surgically repaired nose or facial burns. But because of its non-airtight seal, the face tent doesn't deliver accurate percentages of oxygen.

Setting up. To set up a face tent, follow these steps:
• Attach the face tent and tubing to the humidification device. Set the gas flow at 10 liters/minute.
• Slip the adjustable strap over the patient's head above the ears and place the tent under the chin. Adjust the headband snugly, but not too tightly, so the tent stays in place at the chin.
• Readjust the flow as necessary to produce a visible mist.

Nursing care. Like the trach collar, this system produces high humidification, possibly leading to heavy condensation in the tubing. To prevent problems, drain the condensate often, following the same steps as for the trach collar.

T tube

Also known as the Briggs adapter, the T tube provides oxygen and humidification to a patient with an endotracheal tube or a tracheostomy who isn't receiving mechanical ventilation. One end of the adapter connects to the tubing that provides humidification, and the other end acts as an extension tubing to help maintain a high oxygen concentration.

The device can deliver oxygen concentrations of 21% to 100%, depending on the nebulizer setting and the length of the extension tubing. Using a Venturi nebulizer and adding extension tubing on the exhalation side of the T tube stabilizes oxygen concentrations at high flow rates. (See *T tube.*)

Setting up. To set up a T tube, follow these steps:
• Attach the T tube and tubing to the humidification device. If heating the humidity, turn on the heating device following the equipment manufacturer's instructions.
• Set the flowmeter at 10 liters/minute.
• Attach the T tube to the distal end of the tracheostomy or endotracheal tube.
• Readjust the flow rate to the desired setting. Make sure that the mist is visible.

Nursing care. Like the trach collar, this system produces high humidification, possibly leading to heavy condensation in the tubing. To prevent problems, drain the condensate often, following the same steps as for the trach collar.

Also as with the trach collar,

when delivering heated humidity, monitor the mist temperature. Over-heated aerosol can cause tracheal or pulmonary irritation or burns.

Humidifiers and nebulizers

Normally, inhaled air is warmed and humidified as it passes through the nose, pharynx, and trachea on its way to the lungs. Delivered oxygen bypasses this process, making it cold, dry, and extremely irritating to mucous membranes. Almost all oxygen delivery systems require supplementary humidification — the addition of water vapor to inspired air. Even with a system that may not — such as the Venturi mask or a nasal cannula delivering a flow rate below 2 liters/minute — humidity will usually be added to the room air.

Several humidification devices are available, each with particular indications, advantages, and disadvantages. (See *Comparing humidifiers*, page 126.) Although these devices use different mechanisms to provide humidification, they all share the same basic purposes:
• to add water vapor to inspired air to make breathing more comfortable
• to heat inspired air to provide adequate humidity at body temperature
• to loosen thick or tenacious secretions
• to reduce irritation and edema of the tracheobronchial tree.

Humidity can be added to inspired gas in two ways: through an in-line device, such as the diffusion head humidifier or the cascade bubble diffusion humidifier, which delivers

EQUIPMENT

T tube

The T tube attaches to a tracheostomy or an endotracheal tube to provide oxygen and humidification.

Female adapter

humidified oxygen directly to the patient, or through a room unit, such as a bedside humidifier, which humidifies room air.

Used to deliver moisture or medication, a nebulizer provides 100% humidity in a fine aerosol mist that can be heated or cooled. Heated mist is commonly indicated for neonates and patients with artificial airways; cool mist, for patients with airway edema resulting from recent extubation, tracheotomy, trauma, or other conditions.

Nebulizers can add moisture directly to the lungs to treat epithelial inflammation, smooth muscle bronchospasm, thickened mucosal secretions, and pulmonary infection. They also can deliver medication to affected areas within the tracheobronchial tree to induce sputum production or anesthetize areas of the respiratory tract.

Available nebulizing units include

Comparing humidifiers

Different types of humidifiers offer different advantages and disadvantages, as shown in the following chart.

TYPE	ADVANTAGES	DISADVANTAGES
Diffusion head	• Easy to use • Inexpensive	• Provides only 20% to 30% humidity at body temperature • Can't be used for patient with bypassed upper airway
Cascade bubble diffusion	• Provides 100% humidity at body temperature • Most effective of all evaporative humidifiers • May be used with oxygen hood or in Isolette	• Temperature control may become defective from constant use. • If correct water level isn't maintained, patient's mucosa can become irritated from breathing hot, dry air.
Bedside	• May be used with all oxygen masks and nasal cannula • Easy to operate • Inexpensive	• Produces humidity inefficiently • Can't be used for patient with bypassed upper airway • May harbor bacteria and molds
Heated vaporizer	• May be used with all oxygen masks and nasal cannula • Easy to operate • Inexpensive	• Can't guarantee amount of humidity delivered • Risk of burn injury if machine is knocked over

the Venturi jet (or large-volume) nebulizer and the ultrasonic nebulizer. (See *Comparing nebulizers.*)

Diffusion head humidifier

The in-line humidifier most commonly used in conjunction with low-flow oxygen delivery systems, this device consists of a water reservoir, a standard flowmeter connection, a diffuser made of porous material, and a small-bore outlet connection. Gas flows down a capillary tube to the base of the water reservoir. There, the porous diffuser fragments the gas flow, allowing it to spread and emerge as multiple bubbles. These bubbles move the surface of the water at the top of the jar, increasing the gas-liquid interface. The greater the number and smaller the size of the bubbles, the greater the gas-liquid interface and the amount of humidity produced. (See *Types of humidifiers,* pages 128 and 129.)

Setting up. To set up a diffusion head humidifier, follow these steps:
• Unscrew the humidifier reservoir and add sterile distilled water to the appropriate level. If using a disposable unit, screw the cap with the extension onto the top of the unit.
• Screw the reservoir back onto the humidifier and attach the flowmeter to the oxygen source.
• Screw the humidifier onto the flowmeter, ensuring a tight seal.
• Set the flowmeter at a rate of 2 liters/minute and assess for gentle bubbling.

Comparing nebulizers

The two basic types of nebulizers — Venturi jet and ultrasonic — have different advantages and disadvantages, as seen in the chart below.

TYPE	ADVANTAGES	DISADVANTAGES
Venturi jet nebulizer	• Provides 100% humidity with cool or heated devices • Provides both oxygen and aerosol therapy • Is useful for long-term therapy	• Nondisposable units increase risk of bacterial growth. • Condensate can collect in large-bore tubing. • If correct water level in reservoir isn't maintained, mucosal irritation can result from breathing hot, dry air. • Infants at increased risk of becoming overhydrated from mist
Ultrasonic nebulizer	• Provides 100% humidity • About 20% of its particles reach the lower airways. • Loosens secretions	• May precipitate bronchospasms in the asthmatic patient • May cause overhydration in infants

• Check the positive pressure release valve by occluding the end valve on the humidifier. The pressure should back up into the humidifier, signalled by a high-pitched whistling sound. If this does not occur, tighten all connections and try again.

• Attach the oxygen delivery device to the humidifier and then to the patient. Adjust the flowmeter to the appropriate oxygen flow rate.

Nursing care. Because this unit provides only 40% to 50% humidity at room temperature (which is only 20% to 30% at body temperature), it won't prevent all water loss from the respiratory tract. Periodically assess the patient's sputum; if too thick, it can hinder mobilization and expectoration. If this occurs, the patient requires a device that can provide higher humidity.

Check the reservoir every 4 hours. If the water level drops too low, empty the remaining water, rinse the jar, and refill it with sterile water. (As the reservoir water level decreases, the evaporation of water in the gas decreases, reducing humidification of the delivered gas.)

Change the humidification system at regular intervals to guard against bacterial growth and invasion. Refer to your hospital's policy for changing and disposing of humidification equipment.

Cascade bubble diffusion humidifier

This device is commonly used to provide optimal humidification in patients receiving mechanical ventilation or using a CPAP mask. It includes a water reservoir, a mesh diffuser, a large-bore inlet and outlet and, usually, an immersion heater.

Gas enters the unit and is directed to the bottom of the water reservoir, where it passes through a plastic grid, creating fine bubbles. The gas flow is then directed across the

Types of humidifiers

Illustrated below are the four basic types of humidifiers you may use.

Diffusion head humidifier
This device provides humidification to patients using a nasal cannula and all oxygen masks, except the Venturi mask.

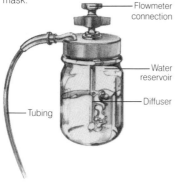

Flowmeter connection

Water reservoir

Diffuser

Tubing

Cascade bubble diffusion humidifier
Commonly used in patients receiving mechanical ventilation or continuous positive airway pressure therapy, the cascade bubble diffusion humidifier delivers 100% humidity at body temperature.

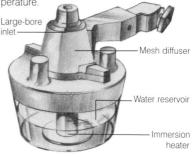

Large-bore inlet

Mesh diffuser

Water reservoir

Immersion heater

water surface, increasing evaporation and, consequently, humidification. The immersion heater warms the vapor to above body temperature.

Setting up. To set up a cascade bubble diffusion humidifier, follow these steps:
• Unscrew the cascade reservoir and add sterile distilled water to the fill line. Screw the top back onto the reservoir.
• Plug in the heater unit, and set the temperature between 95° F (35° C) and 100.4° F (38° C).
• Check the in-line thermometer to ensure that the desired temperature has been reached. If an in-line thermometer isn't available, check the ventilator for a thermometer located inside the machine. On this type of thermometer, a reading of

slightly less than body temperature is usually sufficient.

Nursing care. Assess the temperature of the inspired gas near the patient's airway every 2 hours when used in critical care and every 4 hours when used in general patient care. If the cascade becomes too hot, drain the water and replace it. Overheated water vapor can cause respiratory tract burns.

Check the reservoir's water level every 2 to 4 hours, and fill as necessary. If the water level falls below the minimum water level mark, humidification will decrease to that of room air.

Be alert for condensation buildup in the tubing, which can result from the very high humidification produced by the cascade. As the temperature drops along the tubing,

Bedside humidifier

An easy-to-use device, the bedside humidifier directly humidifies room air. It is commonly used for patients with a nasal cannula or Venturi mask without a humidification source.

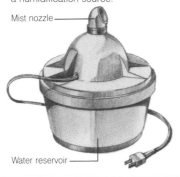

Mist nozzle

Water reservoir

Heated vaporizer

Like the bedside humidifier, the heated vaporizer provides direct humidification to room air. Unlike the bedside humidifier, it does so by heating the water in the reservoir.

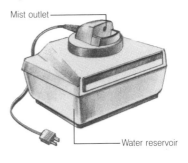

Mist outlet

Water reservoir

the humidity condenses in the tube and can obstruct gas flow. (For this reason, always use large-bore tubing with a heated unit.) Check the tubing frequently and empty the condensate as necessary so it cannot drain into the patient's respiratory tract, harbor and grow potentially dangerous organisms, or obstruct dependent sections of tubing. To do so, disconnect the tubing, drain the condensate into a container, and dispose of it properly. Never drain the condensate into the humidification system or the patient.

Regularly change the cascade according to your hospital's policy. After discontinuing humidification therapy, clean or dispose of all equipment properly.

Bedside humidifier

Used to deliver humidified air to the room atmosphere, the bedside humidifier is especially useful for patients not receiving in-line humidification during oxygen therapy. In this unit, a spinning disk draws water from the water reservoir and propels it against a baffle located in the dome of the unit. When the water strikes the baffle it is fragmented, increasing the surface area exposed to air and increasing evaporation. A motor-driven fan then creates an airflow that disperses a mist out into the room. The mist evaporates, increasing the room's relative humidity.

Setting up. To set up a bedside humidifier, you should follow these steps:

• Open the reservoir and add sterile distilled water to the fill line; close the reservoir.

• Keep all room windows and doors closed tightly to maintain adequate humidification.

• Plug the unit into the electrical outlet.

• Direct the nozzle away from the patient's face, but toward the patient for effective treatment.

• Look for a fine mist emitting from the unit's nozzle, indicating proper operation.

Nursing care. Check the unit every 4 hours for proper operation, and the water level every 8 hours. When refilling, unplug the unit, discard any old water, wipe with a disinfectant, rinse the reservoir container, and refill with sterile distilled water as necessary. Proper cleaning and refilling with sterile water can reduce the potential for bacterial growth. Replace the unit every 7 days and send used units for proper decontamination.

Because this unit doesn't deliver a precise amount of humidification, assess the patient regularly to determine the effectiveness of therapy. Ask him if he feels he has improved and evaluate his sputum.

Instruct a patient using the unit at home to fill it with plain tap water and to periodically use sterile distilled water to prevent mineral buildup. Also explain that running white vinegar through the unit will help clean it, prevent bacterial buildup, and dissolve deposits.

Heated vaporizer

In this unit, consisting of a large water reservoir with an immersion heater, water is drawn into the heating column to produce a mist of steam. When released in the room air, the steam increases the relative humidity. The heated vaporizer is used less commonly than the bedside humidifier, because the risk of

burns from spilling the heated water outweighs the benefits of the increased humidity, especially when the bedside unit provides similar humidification more safely.

Setting up. To set up a heated vaporizer, follow these steps:

• Remove the top and fill the reservoir to the fill line with tap water. Replace the top securely.

• Place the vaporizer about 4′ from the patient, directing the steam toward but not directly onto the patient.

• Plug the unit into an electrical outlet. Steam should rise from the unit into the air.

• Close all windows and doors to maintain adequate humidification.

Nursing care. To avoid hot water burns, place the unit in a spot where it can't be knocked over. This is especially important if children will be in the room.

Check the unit every 4 hours for proper functioning. If steam production seems insufficient, unplug the unit and add a small amount of baking soda to the water. If steam production is excessive, unplug the unit, discard the water, and refill with half distilled water and half tap water, or clean the unit well.

Check the water level in the unit every 8 hours. To refill, unplug the unit, discard any old water, wipe with a disinfectant, rinse the reservoir container, and refill with tap water as necessary.

Like the bedside humidifier, this unit doesn't deliver a precise amount of humidification, so you need to assess the patient regularly by asking if he's feeling better and by examining his sputum.

Rinse the unit with bleach and water every 5 days. Running white vinegar through the unit will also help to clean it as well as to prevent bacterial buildup and dissolve any deposits.

Venturi jet nebulizer

In the Venturi jet nebulizer, the medication or liquid to be delivered is drawn out of a reservoir through a capillary tube. As the fluid enters the high-velocity gas flow, it breaks down into a vast number of aerosol particles. This spray is directed to the baffle, creating a secondary spray that is then directed to the patient. The amount of aerosol produced depends on the gas velocity through the Venturi jet and on the ratio of gas to liquid flow. (See *Venturi jet nebulizer.*)

Setting up. To set up a Venturi jet nebulizer, follow these steps:
• Unscrew the water chamber and fill to the appropriate level with sterile distilled water.
• If ordered, attach the heating device. If possible, use an in-line thermometer beyond the outlet port to monitor the actual temperature of the inhaled gas as close as possible to the patient.
• Attach the flowmeter to the oxygen source, and attach the nebulizer to the flowmeter. Set the flowmeter at 10 to 14 liters/minute. (Large-volume nebulizers require a flow of at least 10 liters/minute for proper operation.)
• Attach the large-bore tubing to the nebulizer and then to the appropriate oxygen delivery device, such as a trach collar or T tube.
• Set the prescribed oxygen concentration.
• Observe the exit port for an ample quantity of mist.

Nursing care. Monitor the temperature for accuracy and instruct the patient to report any excess warmth

Venturi jet nebulizer

The large-volume Venturi jet nebulizer supplies cool or heated moisture to a patient whose upper airway has been bypassed by endotracheal intubation or a tracheostomy, or who has recently been extubated.

Flowmeter adjustment

Outlet port

Heating device

Water reservoir

or discomfort. When turning off the flowmeter, also turn off the heating element to avoid burning the patient.

Use an oxygen analyzer to periodically check the concentration of the oxygen coming from the flowmeter through the nebulizer.

Check the tubing at least every 2 hours to prevent a buildup of water caused by deposits of particles. Such a buildup can adversely affect nebulizer function. If the nebulization is heated, check the tubing more frequently. Empty any excess water into a sink, bucket, or plastic-lined basket—do not put it back into the reservoir.

Ultrasonic nebulizer

The ultrasonic nebulizer uses high-frequency sound waves to create an aerosol mist.

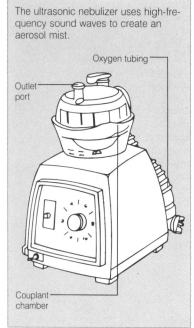

Oxygen tubing

Outlet port

Couplant chamber

Every 4 hours during continuous therapy (more frequently if the unit is heated), check the unit for proper functioning. If necessary, empty the remaining water from the reservoir, rinse the jar thoroughly, and refill with sterile distilled water.

Encourage the patient to frequently cough and breathe deeply to expectorate secretions.

Change the nebulizer every 48 hours and have the unit sterilized, or discard disposable units.

Ultrasonic nebulizer

This device uses high-frequency sound waves to produce an aerosol mist. (See *Ultrasonic nebulizer*.) A piezoelectric transducer creates

the sound waves, which travel to a central focal point in the nebulizer reservoir, where they break up the water into fine particles. The small particle size facilitates their distribution into peripheral lung areas. Adaptable for both continuous and intermittent therapy, the ultrasonic nebulizer is especially useful in treating seriously dehydrated patients with dry, inflamed respiratory mucosa and patients with thick, tenacious secretions, such as occurs in severe bronchitis or cystic fibrosis.

Setting up. Equipment setup varies slightly for intermittent or continuous nebulizer therapy.

To set up the equipment for *intermittent use*, follow these steps:
• Place the unit on a stand or other level surface, and plug the power cord into an electrical outlet.
• Fill the couplant chamber with tap water to the fill line.
• Fill the nebulizer chamber with sterile distilled water or another sterile solution to be nebulized.
• Connect the nebulizer chamber to the gas flow outlet and attach the large-bore tubing to the nebulizer chamber outlet. Then connect the other end of the large-bore tubing to the oxygen delivery device, such as a face mask or T tube.
• Place the delivery device on the patient and tell him to breathe through his mouth. To promote even aerosol distribution throughout the peripheral lung areas, instruct the patient to take a deep breath every few seconds and hold it briefly at the end of inspiration, and then to exhale slowly.
• Increase the ultrasonic output to a level that the patient can tolerate easily.
• Continue the therapy for 10 to 15 minutes. After completing the treat-

ment, empty the nebulizer chamber and thoroughly rinse and dry all equipment.

To set up an ultrasonic nebulizer for *continuous use*, follow these steps:

• Set up the unit and fill its couplant chamber as described above.

• Fill the sterile supply bottle with the desired sterile solution. If using a disposable sterile water container, spike the container, hang it, and attach the container to the nebulizer. If using a continuous-feed system, hang the large-volume bag of sterile distilled water on the hook provided on the nebulizer stand.

• Attach the tubing from the nebulizer bottle to the bag, open the clamp on the tubing, and allow the sterile distilled water to flow into the nebulizer bottle.

• Attach the nebulizer chamber to the gas flow outlet.

• Attach the large-bore tubing to the nebulizer chamber outlet and connect the other end of the large-bore tubing to the oxygen delivery device, such as a face mask, face tent, croup tent, or mist tent.

• Turn on the machine and observe for misting from the outflow port. If using a tent, allow some time for the mist to flush the tent.

Nursing care. Care measures during ultrasonic nebulizer therapy also vary depending on whether therapy is intermittent or continuous.

If your patient is receiving *intermittent therapy,* remain with him during treatment and observe for bronchospasm, dyspnea, and tachycardia. Monitor vital signs and auscultate breath sounds before and after the treatment. Compare posttreatment and pretreatment findings to determine the effectiveness of therapy.

Instruct the patient to breathe

deeply and cough periodically. Note the volume and characteristics of any sputum produced. Suction the patient as necessary, continually monitoring his response.

If your patient is receiving *continuous therapy,* monitor vital signs and auscultate breath sounds at least every 4 hours during treatment. Note any changes in the patient's condition.

Encourage the patient to frequently cough and breathe deeply to enhance sputum expectoration.

Because the risk of bronchospasm and overhydration increases when the ultrasonic nebulizer is used continuously, closely monitor the patient for coughing spasms and wheezing during therapy.

Check the water level every 4 hours. If the water level drops below the top of the transducer, the equipment can overheat and sustain permanent damage.

Pediatric oxygen systems

A child requiring oxygen therapy may be too young to understand its importance and to comply with treatment. Thus, a young child commonly is placed inside an oxygen delivery system to ensure that the oxygen delivery device remains in place throughout the course of treatment. Such systems, which provide an oxygen-rich environment for the child, include the croup tent, oxygen hood, and Isolette. (For more information, see *Pediatric oxygen and humidification devices,* page 134.)

Indicated for children with acute or chronic respiratory disorders, such as croup, asthma, pneumonia, epiglottitis, bronchiolitis, and bron-

Pediatric oxygen and humidification devices

The following chart examines the advantages and disadvantages of devices that deliver oxygen and humidification to children.

TYPE	ADVANTAGES	DISADVANTAGES
Croup tent	• Delivers high humidity and aerosolized therapy • Can be used with oxygen or compressed air • Allows child to move freely • Canopy is disposable.	• Opening tent reduces oxygen concentration; requires 15 to 20 minutes for concentration to return • Ice and water reservoirs must be filled frequently. • System isolates child and increases anxiety. • Difficult to achieve a significant FIO_2 increase • Can decrease body temperature
Oxygen hood	• Enclosed and compact • Provides more precise oxygen concentration than Isolette can by itself • Provides access to infant's lower torso while upper torso remains inside the hood • Functions as a high-flow system when connected to a Venturi delivery system • Can deliver high humidity, either cool or heated	• Can irritate skin • Must remove infant from hood for feeding • An active infant can move out from under the hood.
Isolette	• Enclosed and compact • Can provide enriched oxygen without restricting the infant	• When used without oxygen hood, can deliver only 40% or 100% oxygen. Also, oxygen concentration can fluctuate, depending on how often the unit is opened.

chitis, these systems can provide oxygen and humidification, reduce edema, and help loosen secretions. They also may be used to provide a warm environment for a neonate who needs to conserve body heat, or a cool environment for a febrile child with slight airway edema.

Because the Isolette is used only in newborn nurseries and neonatal intensive care units—two specialized areas of nursing—it isn't discussed in detail.

Croup tent

Also known as a Croupette, the croup tent is designed to provide a cool, high-humidity atmosphere for a child with croup, bronchitis, or pneumonia. It uses a nebulizer to produce aerosol for evaporation within the tent. An electric cooler or an ice chamber cools the oxygen or compressed air before it flows into the tent. (See *Croup tent.*)

Setting up. To set up a croup tent, follow these steps:
• If oxygen is being delivered, post oxygen precaution signs outside the room and above the child's bed. Explain oxygen precautions to all persons who enter the room.
• Assemble the unit and mount it on

Croup tent

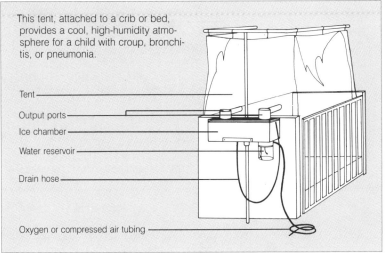

This tent, attached to a crib or bed, provides a cool, high-humidity atmosphere for a child with croup, bronchitis, or pneumonia.

Tent

Output ports

Ice chamber

Water reservoir

Drain hose

Oxygen or compressed air tubing

the back of the bed or crib. Attach the canopy to the unit and position it over the bed. Attach the plastic tent to the overhead frame.

• Fill the reservoir jar with sterile distilled water to the fill line, then fill the ice chamber or turn on the refrigeration unit.

• Plug the cord into an electrical outlet.

• Set the flow-through nebulizer to at least 10 liters/minute, or turn on the air compressor. Observe for a fine mist entering the tent. Flush the tent for a few minutes before placing the child inside.

• For maximum benefit, position the child in a sitting position—using an infant seat, if possible.

• Tuck the sides of the plastic tent under the mattress edges. To seal against leaks, fold a sheet, place it over the front section of the tent, and tuck the ends under the mattress edges.

• After discontinuing therapy, follow your hospital's guidelines for cleaning or disposing of equipment.

Nursing care. Evaluate the effectiveness of therapy by monitoring the child's respiratory status frequently, according to his condition. Also check the child's temperature every 4 hours; the cool atmosphere can decrease body temperature. Use a bath blanket as the bottom bed sheet to absorb excess moisture, and change the child's pajamas or gown as often as needed to keep him warm and dry.

Keep in mind that a child is at particular risk for fluid overload stemming from the high humidification. Monitor daily weight, intake and output, and breath sounds and report any changes to the doctor.

If oxygen is being administered, check the oxygen concentration every 4 hours. Use an oxygen ana-

Oxygen hood

The oxygen hood delivers oxygen and humidification to neonates and infants.

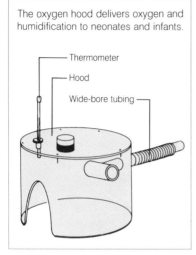

Thermometer

Hood

Wide-bore tubing

lyzer to ensure accurate readings. Open the tent as infrequently as possible; each time the tent is opened, the oxygen level drops — possibly to nearly that of room air — and may not be reestablished for 15 to 20 minutes.

To reduce the risk of fire, keep all battery-operated or electrical toys outside of the tent, particularly when oxygen is being delivered, and follow other oxygen safety measures.

Also check the reservoir every 4 hours. If you need to refill it, remove the jar and pour out any remaining water. Rinse the jar thoroughly and refill with sterile distilled water.

During therapy, give the child constant support and reassurance to help decrease his anxiety and ensure maximum therapeutic benefit. Approach the child and his parents or other caregivers in a calm, reas-

suring manner to inspire their confidence and trust. If possible, have others bring in a security object — such as a favorite doll or blanket — to help decrease the child's anxiety and divert his attention from the isolation of tent therapy.

Oxygen hood

Combining an oxygen source with either a humidifier or a nebulizer, the oxygen hood provides oxygen and humidification to neonates and infants. The hood allows delivery of up to 100% oxygen. (See *Oxygen hood.*)

Setting up. To set up an oxygen hood, first set up the oxygen unit and the humidifier or nebulizer device as described above. Then follow these steps:
• Attach the large-bore tubing to the oxygen hood.
• Place the hood over the child's head and pad it with a towel or foam rubber to maximize comfort and protect against injury.
• Set the prescribed liter flow of oxygen. Make sure that the gas flow is not aimed directly onto the child.
• After discontinuing therapy, send the equipment to the proper department for disinfection.

Nursing care. Continually monitor the child's respiratory status and vital signs to evaluate the effectiveness of therapy. Also monitor for signs of fluid overload; a neonate or infant is at particular risk when using a nebulizer system.

Also monitor the child's ABG values to ensure that arterial oxygen concentrations remain within a normal range. Excessive oxygen concentrations can cause retrolental fibroplasia, possibly leading to blindness.

Check the humidifier or nebulizer

every 4 hours and refill as needed. Also check the tubing and hood every 2 hours for condensation buildup. If this occurs, empty the condensate away from both the child and the humidification device.

When using a heated nebulizer, check the temperature in the hood every 4 hours to ensure that it remains between 96° and 98° F (35.6° and 36.7° C).

Suggested readings

Blodgett, D. *Manual of Respiratory Care Procedures,* 2nd ed. Philadelphia: J.B. Lippincott Co., 1987.

Brunner, L., and Suddarth, D. *Textbook of Medical-Surgical Nursing,* 6th ed. Philadelphia: J.B. Lippincott Co., 1987.

Clinician's Guide to Scoop Transtracheal Oxygen Therapy. Denver: Transtracheal Systems.

Hoffman, L.A., et al. "Patient Response to Transtracheal Oxygen Delivery," *American Review of Respiratory Disease* 135(1):153-56, January 1987.

Kinney, M.R., et al. *AACN'S Clinical Reference for Critical-Care Nursing,* 2nd ed. New York: McGraw-Hill Book Co., 1988.

Wesmiller, S.W., et al. "Understanding Transtracheal Oxygen Delivery," *Nursing89* 19(12):43-47, December 1989.

5

MECHANICAL VENTILATION

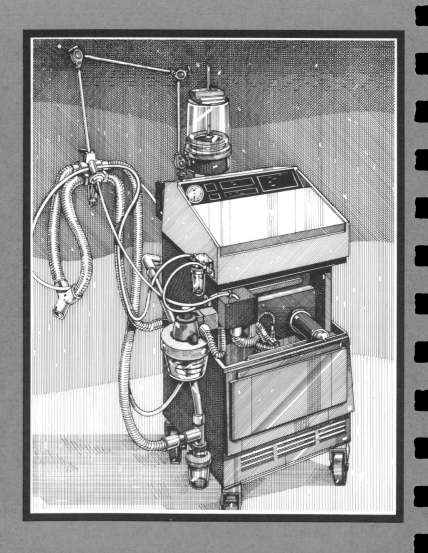

When a patient suffers respiratory failure, mechanical ventilation can supply oxygen, reduce dyspnea, and allow fatigued ventilatory muscles to rest and become reconditioned. Mechanical ventilation does this by artificially controlling or supporting the patient's breathing efforts. Because it also supports spontaneous breathing, mechanical ventilation allows healing to take place until normal respiratory function can resume.

To give the best possible care to a patient receiving such therapy, you need to understand how mechanical ventilation works and how to provide it. This chapter will help you gain that understanding. It describes ventilator types and ventilation modes, as well as the two main adjuncts to ventilator therapy: continuous positive airway pressure (CPAP) and positive end-expiratory pressure (PEEP). The chapter also covers nursing care, including how to manage common complications and how to prepare the patient and his family for home ventilator therapy. Finally, you'll review when and how to wean your patient from a ventilator and when to discontinue weaning.

Basics of mechanical ventilation

Ventilators come in a variety of types, including volume-cycled and pressure-cycled. And ventilation can be delivered in a variety of modes, such as continuous mandatory and intermittent mandatory. A mode, as you may know, determines how much inspiratory effort a patient will need to trigger a ventilation cycle from the machine. Both the type and mode you'll use will depend on your patient's condition.

Certain patients may also require adjunct therapy, such as CPAP or PEEP, to prevent alveolar collapse. Both types of therapy deliver pressure at the end of expiration—CPAP for patients breathing spontaneously, PEEP for patients receiving machined-delivered breaths. (See *Understanding respiratory cycles with PEEP*, page 140.)

Indications

A patient needs mechanical ventilation when he can't generate spontaneous respirations or when his respirations aren't sufficient to expand his chest and deliver oxygenated gas to his lungs. Thus, a doctor will usually base his decision to initiate mechanical ventilation on such signs as accessory muscle use, labored breathing, rapid respiratory rate (more than 25 breaths/minute), and airway obstruction. Typically, he won't wait for the results of arterial blood gas (ABG) analysis and pulmonary function tests.

Two types of disorders—gas exchange and extrapulmonary—call for mechanical ventilation. In gas exchange disorders, mechanical ventilation aims to increase oxygenation, whereas in extrapulmonary disorders, it helps control or support respiratory mechanics.

Gas exchange disorders. Disorders altering gas exchange affect ventilation, perfusion, or both. A respiratory infection, for instance, fills alveoli with secretions, interfering with ventilation. Pulmonary emboli reduce the amount of blood available for diffusion at the alveolocapillary membrane. And adult respiratory distress syndrome (ARDS) disrupts both ventilation and perfusion

Understanding respiratory cycles with PEEP

A mechanical ventilator simulates the normal bellows action of the lungs. By changing the timing of the phases of inspiration and expiration, the ventilator can establish a pattern to meet each patient's needs. This graph shows what happens when a patient receives a machine-delivered breath in combination with positive end-expiratory pressure (PEEP).

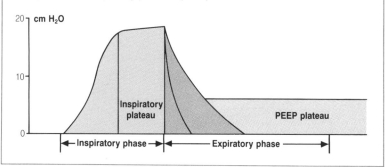

while also causing changes in the alveolocapillary space that impede diffusion across the membrane even if ventilation and perfusion remain adequate. In these situations, mechanical ventilation increases the oxygen available (especially to areas least affected by infection) while the patient receives treatment for the underlying problem.

Extrapulmonary disorders. Instead of directly affecting ventilation or perfusion, extrapulmonary disorders interfere with normal neurologic or neuromuscular mechanics. Central nervous system (CNS) disorders—a brain stem injury, for instance—disrupt neural control of respiration. Neuromuscular diseases, such as Guillain-Barré syndrome, stop stimuli from being transmitted to the respiratory muscles. Flail chest and other musculoskeletal disorders lower tidal volume by keeping the chest from expanding adequately. In these situations, mechanical ventilation controls or

supports respiratory mechanics.

Types of ventilators

Ventilators come in four basic types: negative-pressure, pressure-cycled, volume-cycled, and high-frequency. Each type is classified according to the mechanism that cycles the ventilator.

Most of the time, you'll work with pressure-cycled or volume-cycled ventilators, but you still should understand how all types work (see *Understanding types of mechanical ventilators,* pages 142 and 143).

Negative-pressure ventilators. The original ventilators, negative-pressure machines work by alternately removing and replacing air from a container that encloses either the entire body, except for the head (the Drinker respirator, or iron lung), or just the front and sides of the chest and upper abdomen (the chest shell). Removing air creates a negative pressure in the chamber that forces the chest wall to expand, pulling air into the lungs. Then the device's diaphragm returns to its normal position, allowing the chest wall to fall and causing exhalation.

Although these machines don't require an artificial airway (an important advantage), they do present several drawbacks. They're noisy and restrictive—especially the iron lung—and they make it difficult to provide nursing care. The chest shell ventilator also makes it difficult to maintain a seal.

Pressure-cycled ventilators. These ventilators stop inspiration when they reach a preset pressure and then allow passive expiration. Used mainly for short-term therapy (less than 24 hours), pressure-cycled ventilators reduce the risk of lung damage from high inspiratory pressure. For this reason, you'll commonly see them used on neonates, who have a smaller lung capacity.

Pressure-cycled ventilators have an important drawback: Because they deliver a preset pressure, airway resistance and poor lung compliance can decrease tidal volume. At the same pressure setting, a patient who has stiff lungs or mucus plugs will receive a smaller tidal volume than a patient who has normal lungs. As with all ventilators, you'll have to monitor a patient with poor lung compliance for signs of inadequate ventilation. You'll also have to watch for indications of excessive pressure, which can cause barotrauma.

Volume-cycled ventilators. The most commonly used ventilators, these machines stop inspiration when they've delivered a preset volume of gas, regardless of the pressure needed to deliver it, and then allow passive expiration. They come with several different settings, features,

and modes. As ordered, you can set the tidal volume, respiratory rate, inspiratory-expiratory (I:E) ratio, and, by adjusting the flow rate, inspiratory time. To maintain an adequate partial pressure of oxygen in arterial blood (PaO_2), you can also set the oxygen concentration—measured as the fraction of inspired oxygen (FIO_2)—anywhere from 0.21 (room air) to 1.0.

Volume-cycled ventilators have several features you won't find on the pressure-cycled models, including an automatic sigh mechanism (usually set to activate one to three times a minute). This mechanism reexpands alveoli to prevent atelectasis. (When a patient is receiving PEEP, you won't see this setting used because it can cause excessively high pressures.) These machines also have pressure limit alarms to alert you to high peak airway pressures, which can cause lung damage. And a high-pressure relief valve on some machines relieves excessive pressure—particularly useful when a high pressure is needed to deliver a preset volume.

Unlike pressure-cycled ventilators, volume-cycled machines deliver adequate tidal volume even when airway resistance increases because of changes in airway pressure or lung compliance. This makes them ideal for patients suffering from ARDS or bronchospasm.

A newer type of volume-cycled ventilator also allows pressure ventilation. This type allows you to choose from several different modes. One model even allows reversal of the I:E ratio with a mode called pressure-controlled inverse ratio ventilation. This mode is used when PEEP alone can't prevent alveolar collapse during expiration. You can

(Text continues on page 144.)

Understanding types of mechanical ventilators

Mechanical ventilators come in a variety of types, each with its own indications, advantages, and disadvantages. Here are some of the more common types of mechanical ventilators and their features.

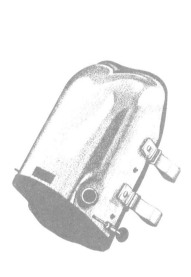

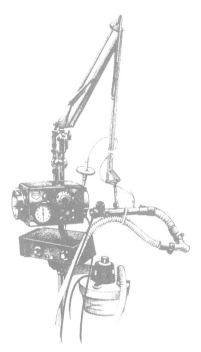

Negative-pressure ventilator (chest shell)
• Creates negative pressure, pulling the thorax outward and pulling air into lungs
• Uses Velcro straps at elbow, hips, and neck to confine negative pressure to chest and abdomen
• Useful for long-term ventilation in patients who have weak respiratory muscles or inadequate respiratory drive
• Allows more freedom of movement than iron lung
• Difficult to seal shell tightly

Pressure-cycled ventilator
• Generates flow until machine reaches a preset pressure
• Used for short-term therapy (less than 24 hours)
• Useful for patients who may suffer lung damage from excessive inspiratory pressure, such as neonates
• Tidal volume varies with airway resistance and lung compliance
• May not adequately ventilate alveoli

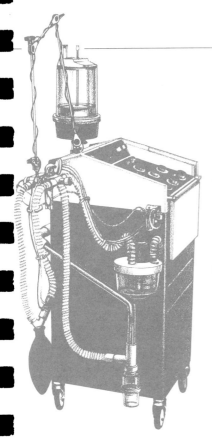

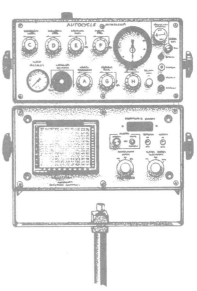

Volume-cycled ventilator
- Most commonly used ventilator
- Delivers preset volume
- Effectively treats respiratory failure in adults by delivering consistent tidal volume despite changes in airway resistance or lung compliance
- Requires regular pressure monitoring to prevent barotrauma

High-frequency jet ventilator
- Delivers 100 to 600 breaths/minute with a tidal volume of only 50 to 400 ml
- Maintains adequate alveolar ventilation with low airway pressure
- Useful for treating tracheoesophageal or bronchopleural fistula, pneumothorax, or pneumomediastinum
- May avert cardiovascular changes and barotrauma in high-risk patients if used early during treatment
- Still experimental

EQUIPMENT

Understanding common volume-cycled ventilators

A look at the control panels of these two volume-cycled ventilators will show you some of their features.

MA-2 + 2
This ventilator can deliver a preset tidal volume. Plus, it has several modes and adjuncts, a sensitivity setting that determines how easily a patient can trigger a breath, and a number of alarms to alert you to various problems.

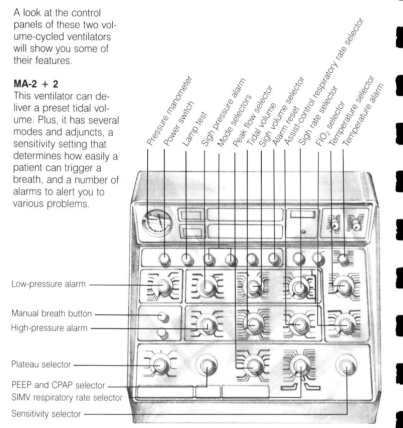

Pressure manometer
Power switch
Lamp test
Sigh pressure alarm
Mode selectors
Peak flow selector
Tidal volume
Sigh volume selector
Alarm reset
Assist-control respiratory rate selector
Sigh rate selector
FIO₂ selector
Temperature selector
Temperature alarm

Low-pressure alarm
Manual breath button
High-pressure alarm
Plateau selector
PEEP and CPAP selector
SIMV respiratory rate selector
Sensitivity selector

set the ratio anywhere from 1:4 to 4:1.

These newer volume-cycled ventilators do have some drawbacks: They require a compressed air source, making them less convenient than other volume-cycled machines, and they cost more than other types of ventilators. (See *Understanding common volume-cycled ventilators*.)

High-frequency ventilators. These ventilators use high respiratory rates (usually four times the normal rate) and small tidal volumes (less than or equal to the patient's dead-space volume) to keep alveoli ventilated. The small tidal volume diminishes the risk of barotrauma and cardiovascular changes.

High-frequency ventilation comes in three varieties:

Siemens-Servo 900C
This newer ventilator has the same features as the MA-2 + 2 and a few others. For instance, it has more ventilation modes and allows reversal of the inspiratory-expiratory (I:E) ratio. It automatically measures the pressure and volume of air the patient receives. And its built-in infant scale lets you more easily adapt the machine to an infant's needs.

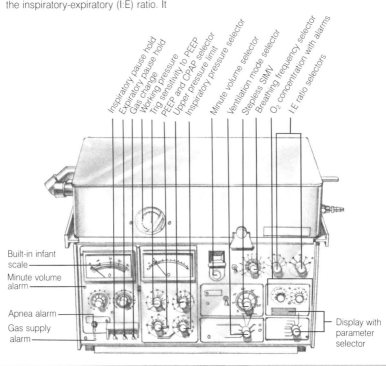

Inspiratory pause hold
Expiratory pause hold
Gas change
Working pressure
Trig sensitivity to PEEP
PEEP and CPAP selector
Upper pressure limit
Inspiratory pressure selector
Minute volume selector
Ventilation mode selector
Stepless SIMV
Breathing frequency selector
O_2 concentration with alarms
I:E ratio selectors

Built-in infant scale
Minute volume alarm
Apnea alarm
Gas supply alarm

Display with parameter selector

• *High-frequency positive-pressure ventilation.* Infrequently used, this type of ventilation generates a breath when a volume of compressed gas is delivered via a pneumatic valve. An angled side arm directs the gas to the patient during inspiration and lets the patient exhale passively. The FIO_2 the patient receives matches that of the compressed gas.

• *High-frequency jet ventilation (HFJV).* In HFJV, gas moves at a pressure of 10 to 50 psi through a fluid or electromechanical control system that has a flow interrupter and an electric timer. Traveling through a transtracheal catheter or the extra lumen of an endotracheal tube, small, pulsed jets of gas with a tidal volume of only 50 to 400 ml enter the patient's airway at a rate of 100 to 600 breaths/minute. The jet stream propels the entrained gas down the trachea, oxygenating the patient, who then exhales passively. The I:E ratio can vary.

You may see HFJV used along with a volume-cycled ventilator set on the CPAP mode. Because HFJV keeps airway pressure low (keeping alveolar distention to a minimum), it increases functional residual capacity (FRC), which stabilizes alveolar ventilation and improves arterial oxygen tension.

Either a cascade humidifier on the volume-cycled ventilator or an infusion of normal saline solution into the endotracheal tube keeps the gas moist. The mixture of entrained gas and jet flow makes the tidal volume difficult to calculate.

• *High-frequency oscillation (HFO).* This type of ventilation vibrates the delivered gas at a rate ranging from 690 to 3,000 cycles per minute. Because HFO delivers limited tidal volumes, it's most suitable for infants with severe neonatal respiratory distress syndrome.

Modes of ventilation

Mechanical ventilation comes in several basic modes, including continuous mandatory ventilation (CMV), assist-control ventilation (ACV), intermittent mandatory ventilation (IMV), synchronized intermittent mandatory ventilation (SIMV), pressure-support ventilation (PSV), pressure-controlled inverse ratio ventilation (PC-IRV), airway pressure release ventilation (APRV), and synchronous independent lung ventilation (SILV). The doctor will choose specific modes based on each patient's condition and ventilatory needs. Each mode ends expiration and signals the machine when to initiate inspiration. (See *Mechanical ventilation modes.*)

Continuous mandatory ventilation. This ventilation mode delivers a preset tidal volume at a set rate, regardless of the patient's attempts to breathe on his own. You'll use CMV for patients with apnea caused by a CNS or neuromuscular dysfunction (such as nerve damage or paralysis, severe brain trauma, Guillain-Barré syndrome, spinal cord injury, and poliomyelitis), a drug overdose, or status asthmaticus.

Because CMV prevents a patient from breathing on his own, it can create anxiety and agitation, causing a conscious or semiconscious patient to fight the ventilator. If the doctor orders a neuromuscular blocker, such as pancuronium, be sure the patient understands the rationale and the drug's paralyzing effects. This mode is available on volume-cycled ventilators.

• *Advantages and disadvantages.* Because it completely controls the patient's breathing, CMV decreases the work of breathing, which decreases his oxygen consumption and carbon dioxide (CO_2) production.

Despite this advantage, CMV also has several drawbacks. It doesn't allow the patient to compensate when his CO_2 level increases. And because the machine, not the patient, does the work of breathing, CMV causes respiratory muscles to atrophy, making it harder to wean the patient from the ventilator.

CMV has adverse cardiovascular effects, too, including decreased venous return and cardiac output caused by iatrogenic alkalemia and increased intrathoracic pressure.

Assist-control ventilation. Used for patients with normal respiratory drive but weak respiratory muscles, ACV augments breathing without completely controlling it. When the patient begins to take a breath,

Mechanical ventilation modes

The pressure waveforms at right show the patterns of common mechanical ventilation modes. Each graph shows the point at which inspiration starts. When applicable, arrows point to the beginning of patient-initiated breaths that trigger the ventilator to deliver a breath. The graphs also show the relative duration of inspiration and expiration. The gray areas indicate inspiration; the blue areas, expiration. The numbers to the left of the graphs indicate pressure in cm H_2O.

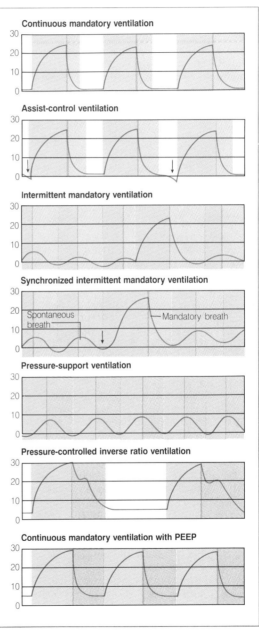

Continuous mandatory ventilation

Assist-control ventilation

Intermittent mandatory ventilation

Synchronized intermittent mandatory ventilation

Spontaneous breath   Mandatory breath

Pressure-support ventilation

Pressure-controlled inverse ratio ventilation

Continuous mandatory ventilation with PEEP

the decrease in pressure triggers ventilation, and the machine delivers the preset tidal volume. When the patient can't breathe on his own, the ventilator takes over, guaranteeing minimum ventilation.

A sensitivity control setting lets you adjust the amount of negative pressure needed for the patient to initiate a ventilation. The less sensitive the machine is to the patient, the greater his work of breathing; the more sensitive, the greater the risk of hyperventilation (especially if the patient breathes rapidly). Usually the pressure is set at -1 to -3 cm H_2O.

Like CMV, this mode is a feature of volume-cycled ventilators.

• *Advantages and disadvantages.* ACV makes weaning easier because it doesn't cause the muscle atrophy that CMV can cause. And ACV lets the patient respond to changes in CO_2 levels. However, this ventilation mode can also cause the same cardiovascular problems as CMV.

Intermittent mandatory ventilation. Used as a means of partial ventilatory support, IMV lets the patient do some of the work of breathing. As in CMV, the patient receives a breath at a preset tidal volume and ventilatory rate, regardless of his efforts. But he can initiate an independent breath between mandatory ventilations, and the machine will deliver humidified, oxygenated gas from a separate circuit to support that breath.

The doctor will usually order the tidal volume set between 10 and 15 ml/kg of the patient's ideal body weight. The rate is set at the lowest level that will let the patient do some of the work of breathing while still maintaining normal ABG and pH levels. If the patient's partial pressure of CO_2 in arterial blood

($PaCO_2$) rises too high, or if his respiratory rate rises above 25 breaths/minute, notify the doctor so he can adjust the rate.

The peak inspiratory pressure limits shouldn't be set higher than 10 cm H_2O above peak inspiratory pressure because of the danger of stacked breaths (a ventilator breath on top of a spontaneous breath). Using a machine with a high-pressure relief valve reduces this risk.

You can use IMV when a patient is on a volume-cycled ventilator.

• *Advantages and disadvantages.* Like ACV, this mode keeps the patient's muscles from atrophying and allows him to respond to changes in CO_2 levels by changing his respiratory rate. It also affords him some control over his breathing, decreasing his anxiety and reducing the need for neuromuscular blockers. Plus, because the machine delivers humidified, oxygenated gas even when the patient initiates his own breaths, all the gas the patient breathes has the same temperature, humidity, and oxygen concentration. Lower intrathoracic pressure also means less risk of the cardiovascular problems associated with CMV and ACV. And patients who use PEEP with IMV have less risk of barotrauma than patients who use PEEP with CMV.

Despite these advantages, IMV is contraindicated in patients whose breathing can suddenly change or stop and those who must keep oxygen consumption low and do only minimal work of breathing.

Synchronized intermittent mandatory ventilation. A variation of IMV, SIMV synchronizes machine-delivered breaths to occur when the patient begins a spontaneous breath. If the patient doesn't breathe within a preset time limit, however, the device delivers a mandatory breath and resets itself to respond to the patient's next spontaneous inspiration.

Like the preceding modes, SIMV is available on volume-cycled ventilators.

• *Advantages and disadvantages.* SIMV has the same advantages as IMV — plus, it's more efficient. However, the time lag in machine-delivered breaths increases the work of breathing, which may pose a problem for some patients.

Pressure-support ventilation. A new ventilation mode, PSV doesn't deliver a preset tidal volume; instead, it supports a spontaneous breath with positive pressure. Because the ventilator delivers positive pressure only when it senses the patient taking a breath on his own, the patient determines the rate. Then the ventilator quickly brings airway pressure up to a preset level. The pressure stays at that level until the ventilator senses the drop in flow rate that signals the end of inspiration.

A patient can't receive pressure support if he's already receiving ACV or CMV. Those two modes deliver a preset tidal volume, something PSV doesn't do. (Of course, using pressure support increases tidal volume.) And in the ACV and CMV modes, the ventilator doesn't wait for the patient to take a spontaneous breath.

Similarly, an apneic patient or a patient with an inadequate respiratory drive can't receive PSV because the patient must be able to initiate a breath for the pressure support to activate. Some ventilators have a built-in backup mode, setting off a "fail to cycle" alarm and providing ventilation if the patient doesn't

breathe. Other machines only set off the alarm if they don't detect a breath.

Pressure support can be delivered along with SIMV, PEEP, or CPAP. When the patient can't provide the required minute ventilation, SIMV supplies that ventilation, and any extra breaths the patient takes get some support from the ventilator.

The PSV mode is available on both the pressure-cycled ventilators and some volume-cycled ventilators.

• *Advantages and disadvantages.* PSV reduces the work of breathing while maintaining respiratory muscle function. Plus, the patient feels more comfortable and less anxious and suffers less dyspnea than with other modes.

However, PSV can cause barotrauma, especially if used in conjunction with PEEP or CPAP. The preset pressure of PSV in addition to the pressure of PEEP or CPAP can damage the lungs and cause adverse hemodynamic effects.

Pressure-controlled inverse ratio ventilation. Patients with severely reduced lung compliance, such as those with ARDS, severe acute lung injury, or neonatal respiratory distress syndrome, can benefit from this experimental mode, which complements, but does not replace, CMV. This mode reverses the normal I:E ratio of 1:2, prolonging inspiration and shortening expiration to a ratio of 4:1. The prolonged ratio gives the patient more oxygen at a lower peak airway pressure.

As mentioned earlier, this mode is available on one model of the volume-cycled ventilators.

• *Advantages and disadvantages.* Because of the decreased peak airway pressure, the risk of bronchopulmonary dysplasia and lung damage (such as barotrauma) decreases. Plus, the prolonged I:E ratio keeps alveoli ventilated longer, and the shorter expiration time decreases the patient's risk of alveolar collapse.

One drawback is that this mode can decrease cardiac output. Remember, too, that the inverse ratio makes the patient uncomfortable. Assess him frequently to see if he needs sedation, hyperventilation, or a neuromuscular blocker.

Airway pressure release ventilation. Indicated for patients with lung injury, this experimental mode simultaneously supports ventilation and delivers CPAP.
• *Advantages and disadvantages.* Research studies show that this mode promotes alveolar ventilation and arterial oxygenation without raising airway pressure above the CPAP level or depressing cardiac function.

Synchronous independent lung ventilation. This mode improves oxygenation for patients with severe pulmonary disease or injury affecting only one lung. In most forms of mechanical ventilation, both lungs receive equal ventilation with a homogeneous distribution of gas, which can cause problems if only one lung needs ventilation. The gas follows the path of least resistance into the healthy lung, which becomes overdistended. That leaves the injured lung without enough gas, leading to a ventilation-perfusion mismatch. SILV helps solve that problem by delivering a different volume of gas to each lung.
• *Advantages and disadvantages.* The patient runs less risk of lung damage from high peak pressures in his uninjured lung and gets the oxygen he needs in the other lung.

However, he'll need a double-lumen endobronchial tube inserted to receive SILV, and the narrow lumina of this tube make suctioning thick secretions difficult. Also, the patient may need sedation to help him cope with the discomfort caused by the size and position of the tube.

Adjuncts to mechanical ventilation

Many patients who use mechanical ventilation require adjunct therapy, such as PEEP or CPAP—both of which keep the alveoli expanded. PEEP and CPAP therapy can help patients who don't have enough surfactant, which normally helps keep alveoli from collapsing. A surfactant deficiency may result from neonatal respiratory distress syndrome, ARDS, smoke inhalation, and lung damage from toxic substances.

The ability to keep alveoli expanded also makes PEEP and CPAP useful for some patients with pulmonary edema. If the alveoli become larger and the amount of fluid stays the same, the area available for gas exchange increases—helping the patient to oxygenate. Some clinicians also think the positive pressure pushes fluid back into the alveolar capillaries. (See *Effects of PEEP and CPAP.*)

Both PEEP and CPAP are contraindicated for patients with untreated hypovolemia caused by hemorrhage; dehydration; neurogenic, anaphylactic, or septic shock; or drug-induced decreased cardiac output or compromised circulation. Because these patients already have compromised circulatory systems, the extra pressure generated by PEEP or CPAP would only aggravate the problem. Similarly, PEEP and CPAP are contraindicated for patients with injury or disease affecting only one

Effects of PEEP and CPAP

These waveforms show you the pressure changes caused by positive end-expiratory pressure (PEEP) and continuous positive airway pressure (CPAP) (I = inspiration; E = expiration). The illustrations below depict the effects of PEEP and CPAP on the alveolus.

Pressure exerted in PEEP and CPAP

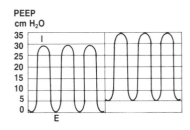

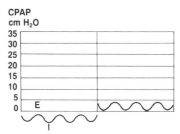

Normal airway pressure baseline of patient on assist-control ventilation (ACV) without PEEP

Normal airway pressure baseline of patient on ACV with PEEP of 5 cm H_2O

Intrathoracic pressure of patient breathing normally

Intrathoracic pressure of patient breathing spontaneously, receiving CPAP of 5 cm H_2O

Effects of PEEP and CPAP on the alveolus

Normal alveolus

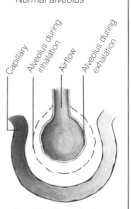

Alveolus with a decreased FRC

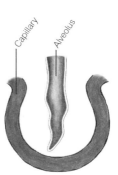

Alveolus expanded using PEEP or CPAP

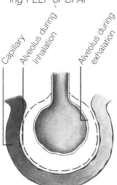

Functional residual capacity (FRC) provides the volume that keeps the alveolus open for gas exchange.

A deflated alveolus provides less area for gas exchange. The dark color indicates a lower PaO_2 in the capillary.

The positive pressure exerted keeps the alveolus expanded, increasing FRC.

lung, because therapy would heighten the difference in blood distribution and ventilation between the two lungs.

These two forms of therapy also are contraindicated for patients with chronic obstructive pulmonary disease (COPD) complicated by hypoxemia, pulmonary hyperinflation, and elevated FRC with increased or normal compliance. High FRC already causes excessive pressure in their lungs, and these adjuncts would only lead to further vascular compression and shunting, venous admixture, and hypoxemia.

Positive end-expiratory pressure. First used in the early 1970s, PEEP lets the patient exhale while maintaining a preset positive pressure at the end of expiration. Maintaining positive airway pressure in the lungs increases FRC and helps inflate and keep open collapsed alveoli, increasing the number available for ventilation. This improves arterial oxygenation, decreases intrapulmonary shunting, and lessens the work of breathing needed to expand collapsed alveoli.
• *Indications.* A doctor may order PEEP for a patient with hypoxemic respiratory failure caused by acute diffuse restrictive lung disease that doesn't respond to supplemental oxygen therapy alone.

Occasionally, you'll use PEEP to increase intrapulmonary pressure in patients with intrathoracic bleeding. The resulting increase in pressure decreases venous return and may lessen bleeding. But decreased venous return also may require giving the patient extra fluids to prevent hypovolemic shock.

Using high-level PEEP in patients with increased intracranial pressure (ICP) raises central venous pressure, which further increases ICP. Such

patients shouldn't receive PEEP unless they also receive adjunct therapy to decrease their CO_2 levels and decrease vasoconstriction.

Patients with bronchopulmonary fistula or those recovering from lung surgery may receive PEEP if they have a chest tube. Monitor these patients carefully for related complications, such as barotrauma.

Continuous positive airway pressure. Used to correct oxygenation failure and to wean patients from mechanical ventilation, CPAP oxygenates by increasing FRC and lung compliance. The patient must be awake and alert, with a PEEP of less than 12 cm H_2O, good tidal volume and vital capacity, a respiratory rate under 24 breaths/minute, normal to low $PaCO_2$, and a normal pH — all indicators that he can maintain the work of breathing. CPAP only works on patients who can breathe spontaneously.

You'll need a continuous flow system to administer CPAP. (Some ventilators have such a system, but you can deliver CPAP without a ventilator.) Intubated patients can receive CPAP through the ventilator's circuitry attached to the endotracheal, nasotracheal, or tracheostomy tube. Other patients can receive CPAP through a tight-fitting, continuous-flow face mask.
• *Indications.* The doctor will order CPAP for a patient who can adequately ventilate but can't effectively oxygenate because of a decreased FRC. Both CPAP and PEEP can help a patient who has secretions blocking his airway or fluid-filled alveoli. Both types of adjunct therapy can also be used to treat refractory hypoxemia resulting from atelectasis — a condition that's common among postoperative patients.

Initiating mechanical ventilation

Usually, a doctor or a respiratory therapist will set up and start mechanical ventilation, but in an emergency, you may need to set up and start the equipment yourself.

Preparing the patient

Before initiating mechanical ventilation, draw a blood sample for baseline ABG analysis. Next, take the patient's baseline vital signs. Also, note his breathing patterns, skin color, and the amount and color of secretions. Assess his level of orientation and responsiveness. The decision to go ahead with mechanical ventilation is usually based on these findings.

Give the patient as much privacy as possible. To reduce his anxiety, explain the procedure step by step, even if he doesn't respond. Tell him why he's being ventilated, describe the sensations he'll feel as the machine controls his breathing, and assure him that a nurse will be nearby at all times.

Place him in semi-Fowler's position, unless contraindicated. This allows his lungs to expand and helps him cough up secretions.

Starting ventilation therapy

To initiate mechanical ventilation:
• Wash your hands and put on gloves.
• If the patient doesn't already have an endotracheal or a tracheostomy tube in place, prepare him for intubation. If he has a tube in place, make sure it's patent. Suction if necessary, and listen for air movement through the tube.

• Auscultate his chest for bilateral breath sounds, and observe for any chest movement.
• Check the manufacturer's instructions for preparing the ventilator. Most guidelines will tell you to bring the ventilator to the bedside, add sterile distilled water to the humidifier, and connect the ventilator to the appropriate gas source.
• Plug the ventilator into the electrical outlet and turn it on.
• Adjust the settings — tidal volume, oxygen concentration, flow rate, and respiratory rate — as ordered. Set all alarms. (See *Responding to ventilator warning signals,* pages 154 and 155.)
• Connect a length of large-bore tubing to the patient's endotracheal or tracheostomy tube, being careful not to dislodge the tube. Make sure you keep the inner lumen of both ends of the tubing sterile.
• Connect the patient to the ventilator and begin mechanical ventilation.

After the patient begins receiving mechanical ventilation, you'll need to assess the adequacy of ventilation and oxygenation. Twenty minutes after beginning ventilation, draw an arterial blood sample for ABG analysis. Compare the results to the baseline values. Also check ABG levels each time the patient's condition or the settings change. The doctor may order the settings adjusted based on these levels.

Maintaining mechanical ventilation

During mechanical ventilation, you'll need to periodically assess the patient; if he's receiving PEEP or

Responding to ventilator warning signals

Most ventilators have alarms to warn you of hazardous situations—for instance, when inspiratory pressure rises too high or drops too low, or when the actual tidal volume varies too much from the set tidal volume. This chart gives you common causes and interventions for three ventilator alarms.

SIGNAL	POSSIBLE CAUSE	INTERVENTIONS
Low-pressure alarm	• Tube disconnected from ventilator	• Reconnect tube to ventilator.
	• Endotracheal tube displaced above vocal cords or tracheostomy tube extubated	• Check tube placement and reposition if needed. If extubation or displacement has occurred, manually ventilate the patient and call the doctor immediately.
	• Leaking tidal volume from low cuff pressure (from an underinflated or ruptured cuff or a leak in the cuff or one-way valve)	• Listen for a whooshing sound around tube, indicating an air leak. If you hear whooshing, check cuff pressure. If you can't maintain pressure, call the doctor; he may need to insert a new tube.
	• Ventilator malfunction	• Disconnect the patient from the ventilator and manually ventilate him if necessary. Get another ventilator.
	• Leak in ventilator circuitry (due to loose connection or hole in tubing, loss of temperature-sensing device, or cracked humidification jar)	• Make sure all connections are intact. Check for holes or leaks in the tubing and replace if necessary. Check the humidification jar; replace it if cracked.
High-pressure alarm	• Increased airway pressure or decreased lung compliance caused by worsening disease	• Auscultate the lungs for evidence of increasing lung consolidation, barotrauma, or wheezing. Call the doctor if indicated.
	• Patient biting on oral endotracheal tube	• If needed, insert a bite guard.
	• Secretions in airway	• Look for secretions in the airway. To remove, suction or have the patient cough.
	• Condensate in large-bore tubing	• Check tubing for condensate. Remove any fluid.
	• Intubation of right mainstem bronchus	• Check tube position. If it has slipped from its original position, call the doctor; he may need to reposition it.
	• Patient coughing, gagging, or attempting to talk	• If the patient is fighting the ventilator in any way, he may need sedation or a neuromuscular blocker, as ordered.
	• Chest wall resistance	• Reposition the patient if his position limits chest expansion. Reassess to see if this has relieved the resistance. If not, administer prescribed analgesic.
	• Failure of high-pressure relief valve	• Have the faulty equipment replaced.
	• Bronchospasm	• Assess the patient for the cause. Report to the doctor and treat as ordered.

Responding to ventilator warning signals *(continued)*

SIGNAL	POSSIBLE CAUSE	INTERVENTIONS
Spirometer or low exhaled volume alarm	• Power interruption • Loose connection or leak in delivery system • Increased airway resistance in a patient on a pressure-cycled ventilator • Spirometer disconnected • Any change that sets off the high- or low-pressure alarm and prevents the full volume of air from being delivered	• Check all electrical connections. • Make sure all connections in the delivery system are secure; check for leaks. • Auscultate his lungs for signs of airway obstruction, barotrauma, or lung consolidation. • Make sure the spirometer is connected. • See interventions for high- and low-pressure alarms.

CPAP, pay special attention to his cardiovascular and ventilatory status so you can prevent or manage problems. You'll also need to check the ventilator to make sure it's functioning correctly.

Proper nursing care also involves using your assessment findings to form nursing diagnoses and implement a care plan. Finally, if the patient will be receiving mechanical ventilation at home, you'll need to prepare him and his family.

Assessing the patient
At the start of ventilation therapy, perform a complete assessment to obtain baseline information. Refer to this information during subsequent assessments so you can note significant changes in the patient's condition.

Neurologic assessment. Check the patient's level of consciousness. Then assess nerve function and innervation, which are key to establishing a regular ventilatory pattern, maintaining protective reflexes in the airway, and responding to

changes in $PaCO_2$ and pH balance. Observe his ability to communicate, and assess his understanding of his problem. (This may give you a chance to relieve some of his fears about mechanical ventilation.) Note any rapid breathing or excessive anxiety; either may signal the need for sedation.

Cardiovascular assessment. The rise in intrapulmonary and intrathoracic pressures caused by mechanical ventilation means you'll need to monitor cardiovascular function carefully. Assess the patient's heart rate and rhythm, peripheral blood pressure, and central pressures. Direct or indirect measurement of cardiac output helps you evaluate effective perfusion to the brain, heart, and kidneys.

Respiratory assessment. Observe the patient's respiratory rate, rhythm, and effort. Assess his use of respiratory muscles and check thoracic shape and excursion. See if his breathing is synchronized with the ventilator. Listen for abnormal and adventitious breath sounds. Observe the type and size of the patient's artificial airway. Then check cuff pressure, looking for any sign of an air leak. Note the amount, color, consistency, translucency, and odor of all secretions. Document how frequently the patient needs suctioning and pulmonary hygiene to keep his airway patent. Changes from this baseline could signal a problem.

Examine chest X-rays and ABG results to help pinpoint changes in the lungs' ability to exchange gas. Check bedside ventilatory measurements — including minute ventilation, respiratory rate, tidal volume, peak inspiratory pressure, plateau pressure, and static compliance — to help determine the success of mechanical ventilation. Also calculate such measurements as alveolar-arterial (A-a) oxygen gradient, intrapulmonary shunt fraction (Qs/Qt), and ratio of dead-space ventilation to total ventilation (Vd/Vt).

Abdominal assessment. Auscultate the abdomen for abnormal bowel sounds, and look for gastric distention. Assess the patient's nutritional status; he must take in enough calories to maintain respiratory muscle strength. If he needs supplemental feedings, be sure to monitor him closely; the metabolic breakdown of these feedings commonly increases CO_2 production.

Measure the amount and pH of gastric secretions and stools, and test both for blood — a sign of occult bleeding. Report any black, tarry stools; they may indicate bleeding in the upper GI tract.

Renal assessment. Monitor the patient's intake and output to check the adequacy of renal and cardiac function. Weigh him daily to detect fluid retention. (You can also use weight as a measure of how well his diet meets his metabolic needs.) Measure his urine specific gravity and osmolality, and test his urine for glucose, acetone, and electrolyte levels. The diagnosis of metabolic and acid-base imbalances depends on measurement of serum osmolality and electrolyte levels.

Mental status. Carefully assess the patient's mental and emotional status. He'll probably be anxious and uncomfortable. Maintaining his sleep-wake cycle will help his orientation and put him more at ease. You can further reduce his anxiety by making sure he has the means to communicate his needs.

Special considerations for PEEP and CPAP patients

A patient receiving PEEP or CPAP requires careful monitoring. Your goals are to achieve or maintain proper oxygenation and to prevent complications.

Adjust PEEP levels, as ordered, in increments of 3 to 5 cm H_2O until the patient's PaO_2 reaches 60 to 70 mm Hg and his FIO_2 drops to 0.5 or less without a significant decrease in cardiac output. You'll usually see PEEP set at 5 to 10 cm H_2O, but you may see it set as high as 40 cm H_2O to reach adequate oxygenation. (See *PEEP: Distinguishing terms.*)

Nursing considerations for a patient receiving CPAP depend on whether the therapy is delivered through an artificial airway or a face mask. An intubated patient receiving CPAP must breathe through a small airway, which increases the work of breathing. This can lead to respiratory fatigue and, in turn, end a weaning attempt. A patient using a face mask will probably need a nasogastric tube to decrease the risk of gastric dilation, vomiting, and aspiration. The face mask also limits your ability to provide upper-airway, mouth, and skin care.

No matter which delivery method is used, most patients can tolerate CPAP for only 12 to 36 hours. If CPAP therapy has been successful, the doctor will discontinue it. If therapy hasn't been successful, the patient may return to positive-pressure ventilation.

Patients receiving PEEP or CPAP need the same body-system assessment as any ventilator patient. Pay special attention to the patient's cardiovascular and ventilatory status to detect early signs of compromise. You'll also need to assess for the particular complications PEEP and CPAP can cause.

Cardiovascular status. Monitor the patient carefully for signs of cardiovascular compromise. Whenever the level of PEEP or CPAP changes, monitor vital signs every 5 minutes for the first 15 minutes, then every 15 minutes until the patient stabilizes, and then hourly to detect any decrease in cardiac output. Report any of the following signs, which may signal hypovolemia: a systolic blood pressure drop of 20 mm Hg or more, increased heart rate, decreased urine output, or altered neurologic status. Make sure arterial blood pressure is at least 70 mm Hg—the level needed to maintain sufficient cerebral, coronary, and renal blood flow. Cardiac monitoring will also help you detect arrhythmias, which increase myocardial oxygen needs and decrease filling time and cardiac output.

Also, monitor hemodynamic measurements closely when the level of PEEP or CPAP is increased or decreased. A decrease, for instance,

PEEP: Distinguishing terms

You'll hear four different terms used to describe the level of positive end-expiratory pressure (PEEP): physiologic PEEP, prophylactic PEEP, super PEEP, and optimal PEEP. Here's what these terms mean.

Physiologic PEEP (3 to 5 cm H_2O) compensates for the lung volume lost when the patient moves from the upright to the supine position.

Prophylactic PEEP (3 to 5 cm H_2O) offsets the loss in functional residual capacity that follows upper abdominal or thoracic surgery.

Super PEEP (above 20 cm H_2O) achieves acceptable oxygenation in critically ill patients with severe, intractable hypoxemia.

Optimal PEEP is the lowest level of PEEP that does not significantly decrease cardiac output while maintaining PaO_2 at or above 60 mm Hg and arterial oxygen saturation at 90% when FIO_2 is at or above 0.5.

increases venous return, which could trigger congestive heart failure (CHF) in a patient prone to it. Continue monitoring for up to an hour afterward, as ordered.

Ventilatory status. Monitor tidal volume, respiratory frequency, minute ventilation, peak and plateau pressures, the level of PEEP or CPAP, and static compliance. You'll also need to check measurements of arterial blood and mixed venous gases, arterial-alveolar oxygen tension ($P[A-a]O_2$) or shunt, and (if available) the arterial minus end tidal carbon dioxide gradient. Consider mixed venous oxygen saturation of 60% normal when the patient has a sufficient hemoglobin level, oxygen delivery, and cardiac output. He should have an A-a oxygen gradient of less than 350.

At least every 2 to 4 hours, assess breath sounds for early signs of pulmonary barotrauma, such as absent breath sounds with decreased pulmonary excursion.

Key measurements. When you monitor the patient's hemodynamic measurements, be sure to include his cardiac output and pulmonary capillary wedge pressure (PCWP). Monitor the patient's heart rate for adequate ventricular filling time. This is determined by a cardiac output of 4 to 8 liters/minute, a cardiac index of 2.5 to 3.5 liters/minute/m^2, and the absence of angina. Measure PCWP at the end of expiration. Although PEEP levels above 15 cm H_2O will raise the PCWP, you can still use this reading as a baseline value to monitor the patient for change.

Also make sure other central pressures are high enough to allow adequate cardiac and urine output (0.5 ml/kg of body weight/hour). Normal right atrial pressure should be 2 to 6 mm Hg; pulmonary artery systolic pressure, 20 to 30 mm Hg; pulmonary artery end-diastolic pressure, 8 to 12 mm Hg; and pulmonary artery wedge pressure, 4 to 12 mm Hg. A mean pulmonary artery pressure of less than 20 mm Hg is normal. A patient with myocardial infarction may need higher central pressures to maintain stroke volume.

Further monitoring. The increase in intrathoracic pressures caused by PEEP and CPAP decreases venous return and, thus, cardiac output. To correct this situation, the doctor may order fluid administration or, sometimes, use of inotropic or pressor agents. Expect to monitor the patient's fluid status using a flow-

directed, balloon-tipped pulmonary artery catheter to prevent fluid overload and increased lung water content.

Watch for signs of pulmonary barotrauma, such as pneumothorax or subcutaneous emphysema. Caused by increased intrapulmonary pressure, the risk of barotrauma increases with PEEP or CPAP levels above 20 cm H_2O. Using IMV rather than CMV or ACV with PEEP decreases this risk.

Checking the ventilator

Besides assessing the patient, you'll need to check the ventilator function and settings every 1 to 2 hours, and as needed to make sure the patient receives the therapy he needs. To check the ventilator, follow these steps:

• Check the ventilator mode and adjunct. Then check tidal volume, respiratory rate, I:E ratio, FIO_2, peak inspiratory pressure, sighs per minute, and temperature settings. Adjust the machine as needed, according to the patient's prescribed therapy.

• Measure the patient's tidal volume, plateau pressure, and static compliance.

• Make sure all alarms are set.

• Check the airway pressure gauge. A sudden change may mean the ventilator needs resetting. Gradually falling pressure may signal a leak in the system; rising pressure, right mainstem bronchus intubation, barotrauma, or the need for suctioning. Report either change to the doctor so he can assess the patient and adjust the ventilator settings, if necessary.

• Monitor exhaled tidal volume with a respirometer to make sure the machine delivers an adequate volume to the patient.

• If the patient is on a ventilator

that heats the airflow, make sure the gauges remain between 95° and 98.6° F (35° and 37° C). If necessary, adjust the temperature of the gas delivered to the patient to within that range.

• Check the water level marker on the humidifier, and refill the reservoir as needed.

• Check for condensation in the large-bore tubing. Empty the water regularly to prevent resistance to airflow and decrease the risk of water aspiration when the patient turns in bed. Disconnect the patient from the ventilator and quickly drain any condensate into a collection container so that you can discard it. Don't empty the condensate into the humidifier; it may be contaminated.

• Make sure all connections are secure.

• Document the steps you've taken on the ventilator checklist according to hospital policy.

Forming nursing diagnoses

The effects of ventilator therapy can frighten a patient, make him uncomfortable, or even threaten his recovery. Depending on how well the patient tolerates therapy, he may encounter problems with nutritional status, fluid volume, gas exchange, airway clearance, physical mobility, skin integrity, verbal communication, or sleep patterns. By using your assessment findings and impressions of the patient, you can form nursing diagnoses that identify such problems or the potential for them. In turn, your nursing diagnoses form the foundation of a nursing care plan to prevent or manage these adverse effects of ventilator therapy.

Altered nutrition: Less than body requirements. Always a potential problem with ventilator patients, this leads to respiratory muscle mass breakdown and can delay weaning. If the patient is NPO for even 1 day, he'll need 4 to 5 days of parenteral nutrition to recoup the loss. The doctor will order high-calorie tube feedings if the patient has an intact, healthy GI tract; if not, the doctor may order total parenteral nutrition (TPN).

Fluid volume deficit. Make sure the patient receives enough fluid to maintain intravascular volume, blood pressure, and cardiac output and to loosen bronchial secretions.

Fluid volume excess. Too much fluid can lead to pulmonary edema and further hamper gas exchange. Monitor your patient's intake and output and weigh him daily to assess fluid status.

Impaired gas exchange. This can happen if the patient's airway becomes blocked. To keep it patent, frequently assess the patient for adequate ventilation using inspection, and assess him more fully every hour using inspection, palpation, percussion, and auscultation. Stimulate coughing by setting the ventilator to deliver two to three sighs each hour. If the patient is on a ventilator that doesn't have a sigh mechanism, use a manual resuscitation bag.

Ineffective airway clearance. Suction your patient to prevent ineffective airway clearance, but only when necessary; suctioning can damage the patient's trachea. After suctioning, be sure to wait at least 15 minutes before disconnecting the patient from the ventilator for weaning, chest physiotherapy, or drawing blood for ABG analysis.

This allows blood gases time to return to their previous levels.

Impaired physical mobility. If the patient needs pancuronium or another neuromuscular blocker, he won't be able to blink. Keep his eyes moist with saline solution; you can also close them with eye patches. Immobility also decreases muscle strength and joint mobility. Begin active and passive range-of-motion exercises as soon as possible. Teach family members how to help the patient perform these exercises. (See *When your patient is receiving pancuronium.*)

Impaired skin integrity. Pressure sores cause pain and increase the risk of infection. You can help prevent these sores by keeping the patient's skin dry, turning him every 2 hours, keeping his sheets dry and wrinkle-free, and using a special bed or mattress, such as a convoluted foam mattress.

Impaired verbal communication. Intubation interferes with speech, making the patient anxious and frustrated. The endotracheal tube passes between the vocal cords, forcing them open. If the patient tries to speak, or even move his lips, his vocal cords reflexively contract around the tube, causing trauma and edema. Give your patient a letter board or a pad of paper and a felt-tipped marker so he can communicate.

Sleep pattern disturbance. This weakens the patient and delays weaning from the mechanical ventilator. In a long-term intensive care unit patient, lack of sleep can even contribute to psychosis. Arrange for uninterrupted sleep periods whenever possible.

Preparing the patient for home care

A stable patient who still needs mechanical ventilation — one with neuromuscular disease or chronic lung disease without systemic complications, for instance — is a candidate for home ventilator therapy. Before discharge, teach him and his caregiver how to manage his care, recognize danger signs, and correct common equipment malfunctions. (See *Managing ventilator problems at home,* page 162.)

Airway assessment. Show the caregiver how to assess the patient's respiratory rate and recognize changes in his breathing pattern — including danger signs, such as shortness of breath and apnea. Then teach the caregiver how to describe the quality and amount of secretions so she can report her findings to the doctor.

Bagging technique. Teach the caregiver the purpose of the appropriate equipment. Then show her how to connect the manual resuscitation bag to the oxygen source and the tracheostomy tube. Make sure she knows how to give the patient oxygen at a comfortable rate.

Sterile suctioning. Teach the caregiver how to suction the patient, and help her select the proper equipment she'll need (catheter, gloves, manual resuscitation bag, and sterile container of saline solution). Stress the importance of proper hand-washing and sterile suctioning technique.

Tracheostomy tube cleaning. Explain to the caregiver the procedure for cleaning the tracheostomy tube, stressing the importance of aseptic technique.

When your patient is receiving pancuronium

When a patient receiving continuous mandatory ventilation fights the ventilator, his doctor may order pancuronium. A neuromuscular blocker, pancuronium inhibits acetylcholine binding at cholinergic nicotinic receptors on skeletal muscle membranes, causing flaccid paralysis. You'll administer it, as ordered, to paralyze the patient temporarily so that he can get the tidal volume he needs.

When you care for a patient who's receiving pancuronium, take these measures:
☐ Always keep emergency resuscitation equipment nearby. If the machine malfunctions, the patient will need manual ventilation.
☐ Keep drugs that reverse the effects of pancuronium – neostigmine and edrophonium – close at hand. Remember, the effects of pancuronium continue for about 90 minutes after the drug has been discontinued.
☐ Because pancuronium doesn't decrease level of consciousness, always announce your presence and explain what you're there to do when you enter the patient's room.
☐ Reassure the patient that the paralysis he's feeling is temporary and an effect of the drug – not a result of his underlying condition – and is actually helping him get the ventilatory assistance he needs.
☐ Inform his friends and family about the effects of pancuronium. Make sure they understand that the patient is fully conscious and can hear what they say to him.
☐ Monitor his vital signs. Pancuronium can cause hypotension and tachycardia.
☐ Regularly moisten his eyes with saline solution to compensate for his temporarily absent blink reflex.
☐ Administer an analgesic, as ordered, if the patient's condition indicates he's in pain.

Tell the caregiver to wash her hands and then to gather the following equipment: gloves, equal parts hydrogen peroxide and saline solution (or other cleaning solution) to clean the cannula and the patient's skin, a brush, pipe cleaners, tracheostomy tape, and sterile 4″ × 4″ gauze pads. An extra sterile tracheostomy tube should always be kept by the patient's bed.

Have the caregiver unwrap the equipment and disconnect the patient from the ventilator. Then tell her to put on the gloves and remove the inner cannula. Describe how to submerge the cannula in the cleaning solution and clean it with the brush and pipe cleaners. Have her hold it to the light to inspect for cleanliness. Stress the importance of monitoring the patient's respiratory status throughout the cleaning procedure.

Next, have the caregiver shake off any extra fluid and reinsert the cannula, locking it into place. Then she can reconnect the patient to the ventilator. After that, she should remove the gauze pad from around the tracheostomy, clean the skin using sterile gauze pads and more of the cleaning solution, and put a new gauze pad around the stoma. Caution the caregiver to change the tracheostomy tape only if another person – even the patient, if he's able – can help. Finally, tell her to discard the used equipment (including gloves) and to record the

Managing ventilator problems at home

A patient's home caregiver must know how to handle certain common ventilator problems. She also must know when to call for emergency help.

Emphasize to the caregiver the importance of remaining calm when a ventilator problem develops. And teach her how to manage the following common problems.

Obstructed tracheostomy tube
• Disconnect the patient from the ventilator.
• Provide oxygen, using a manual resuscitation bag.
• Suction him.
• Irrigate with saline solution, if necessary.
• Reconnect him to the ventilator, and assess his respiratory status.
• If he's still in respiratory distress, call for an ambulance.

Water in the tubing
• Disconnect the tubing from the ventilator.
• Empty the water from the tubing, and reconnect the tubing to the ventilator.

Incorrect cuff pressure
• Inflate or deflate the cuff to the correct pressure.

condition of the skin around the stoma.

After you've gone over these steps with the caregiver, make sure she understands the danger of the outer cannula coming out of the tracheostomy site. Teach her how to insert the new tracheostomy tube and tie it securely and how to assess the patient's respiratory status. Tell her to call the home health nurse or the doctor if any problems develop.

Preventing complications

Mechanical ventilation affects many body systems, not just the lungs. And it can cause complications, even when the equipment works and is used properly. When the equipment malfunctions or isn't set up correctly, the risk of injury skyrockets. Mechanical ventilation can produce both physical and psychological complications. Some of the physical problems — tension pneumothorax, for example — can be life-threatening.

Mechanical malfunctions
Though common, mechanical malfunctions are preventable or reversible. You can help avoid many malfunctions by familiarizing yourself with the ventilator and its alarm system and by making sure the alarms always stay on.

The most common causes of mechanical malfunctions include:
• failure to set alarms
• failure to stabilize ventilator tubing, resulting in kinks or accidental extubation
• electrical failure
• incorrect temperature settings (too high a setting causes tracheobronchial burns; too low, inadequate humidification, bronchospasm, and mucus plugs)
• malfunction of the fail-safe valve, preventing the patient from exhaling.

In any of these situations, an unparalyzed, arousable patient will show obvious signs of respiratory distress — gasping, tachypnea, tachycardia, and asynchronous breathing. If you detect any of these signs, remove the patient from the ventilator and manually ventilate him. To provide positive-pressure ventilation, use a self-inflating manual resuscitation bag that supplies enough oxygen and PEEP. Add a PEEP attachment to the manual resuscitation bag if the patient needs to receive PEEP greater than 10 cm H_2O.

Physical complications

Assess the patient carefully to detect physical complications that can result from mechanical ventilation. These include airway malfunction, airway trauma, acid-base balance alterations, arrhythmias, asynchronous breathing, atelectasis, barotrauma, decreased venous return, GI alterations, infection, and oxygen toxicity.

Airway malfunction. A common complication, airway malfunction can result from an obstruction (such as a mucus plug), cuff underinflation or rupture, extubation or incorrect tube placement, or disconnection from the ventilator.

Assess the patient frequently for signs of an airway obstruction. Use suction to remove mucus accumulation; if necessary, instill saline solution to make thick secretions easier to suction.

Listen for airway leaks as the ventilator cycles to detect cuff underinflation or rupture; a whooshing sound at the patient's mouth indicates that gas is leaking past the cuff. This may decrease the amount of oxygen the patient receives and prevent PEEP or CPAP from working effectively.

Auscultate breath sounds to make sure the tube is in place. If you don't hear breath sounds on both sides of the chest, the tube may be too far above or too close to the carina or blocking a primary bronchus and a lung. Measure the length

of the tube from its tip to the patient's lips to determine if the tube has moved farther into the lungs. If the tube is too close to the carina or in the right mainstem bronchus, deflate the cuff, withdraw the tube 1 to 2 cm, auscultate again, and, when you hear breath sounds in both lungs, reinflate the cuff. Check the tape to see if it may have loosened enough to let the tube slip out of position (the weight of the ventilator tubing may have pulled the patient's tube out of place). If the tube has slipped, notify the doctor. Don't automatically retape the tube; each time you retape, the movement of the endotracheal tube traumatizes the vocal cords. Only retape if the skin is irritated or the tape is soiled or loose enough to let the tube be dislodged again.

Reposition the tube once every 8 hours to the other side of the patient's mouth. Then make sure the connection between the large-bore tubing and the patient's tube is secure.

Airway trauma. This complication can occur during intubation, extubation, or maintenance. The longer an artificial airway remains in place, the greater the risk. Two-thirds of patients who have an artificial airway in place for more than 30 days develop some form of injury.

Several factors increase that risk, including traumatic intubation, pulling or rubbing of the tube, the presence of nasogastric or duodenal tubes, and excessive cuff pressure. Even trying to speak with the airway in place can cause injury.

The patient's physical state can increase the chance of injury, too. Edema formation, an upper respiratory obstruction, dehydration, too much secretion in the airway, and recent surgery of the neck all increase the risk of airway trauma. And a patient in an impaired metabolic state won't recover from injury as quickly.

Some patients don't tolerate intubation well, including those with anatomic abnormalities in their airways, elderly patients, and pediatric and female patients, who commonly have thin tracheal linings.

To reduce the risk of injury, use the right size tube and give meticulous tube care. Make sure the cuff is not overinflated. A pressure of between 15 and 22 mm Hg, or use of the minimal occlusive leak technique, helps prevent injury.

Alterations in acid-base balance.
Mechanical ventilation can cause an increase or decrease in $PaCO_2$. If the patient can't breathe deeply or fast enough, he can't release enough CO_2. Levels will build up in his blood, resulting in hypercapnia, which increases the concentration of hydrogen ions, decreases pH, and causes respiratory acidosis. Vasodilation results, increasing cerebral blood flow and pressure in the brain, which can cause lethargy, possibly progressing to coma. To correct vasodilation, increase ventilation by increasing the respiratory rate or tidal volume, as ordered.

The opposite extreme, respiratory alkalosis, results from hyperventilation. The patient exhales too much CO_2, decreasing $PaCO_2$ and increasing blood pH. Too rapid a decrease causes vasoconstriction, preventing enough blood from getting to the brain and resulting in seizures and coma. The hypokalemia that accompanies alkalosis also increases the risk of tetany and arrhythmias. The resulting shift to the left of the oxygen-hemoglobin curve increases hemoglobin's affinity for oxygen, resulting in tissue hypoxia. This

prevents the patient from being weaned from mechanical ventilation. To correct the problem, decrease the respiratory rate or tidal volume (if it's too high), or increase the length of tubing on the ventilator to increase mechanical dead space, as ordered.

Arrhythmias. Arrhythmias may develop in acute care patients on mechanical ventilation who are at risk of developing metabolic alterations. The stress that ventilator therapy places on the cardiovascular system forces the heart to work harder, increasing myocardial oxygen consumption. When the heart can't get enough oxygen, cardiac output decreases and myocardial hypoxia and acidemia result, possibly leading to arrhythmias. For patients with preexisting coronary artery disease and hypoxemia, the risk of ventricular arrhythmias increases even more.

Continuous cardiac monitoring of these high-risk patients lets you detect arrhythmias. Treating the underlying problem should correct the pattern, or the doctor may order an antiarrhythmic to treat a life-threatening arrhythmia.

Asynchronous breathing. This complication occurs when the patient tries to breathe between or against the ventilator-delivered breaths. Several factors can cause asynchronous breathing. The patient's own anxiety may lead him to try to breathe on his own. He may have hypoxemia, acidosis, or a partially obstructed airway. Or the ventilator may have been programmed or set up incorrectly.

Whatever the cause, fighting the ventilator leads to stacked breathing, which can increase intrapulmonary pressure and cause air hunger. If you see signs of air hunger, remove the patient from the ventilator, manually ventilate him, and assess his airway for patency and his ability to be ventilated. Check his vital signs, breath sounds, and hemodynamic measurements. Suction his airway to remove any obstructions. Draw an arterial blood sample for ABG analysis, and adjust ventilatory support as needed. To keep the patient calm, reassure him that you know he's uncomfortable and that you'll stay with him.

If you can't calm the patient and his air hunger continues despite your interventions, he may need sedation. Expect to administer a neuromuscular blocking agent, as ordered, only if all other attempts to stop asynchronous breathing fail.

Atelectasis. Lobar or segmental atelectasis refers to a collapse of lung tissue that prevents gas exchange during respiration. (See *Understanding atelectasis,* pages 166 and 167.) Possible causes of this complication include tidal volumes too small to inflate alveoli, occluded airways, inadequately humidified gas that can lead to thick mucus, insufficient pulmonary hygiene, failure to aspirate the trachea, and infrequent position changes.

To detect atelectasis, monitor the patient for low-grade fever (usually less than 101° F [38.3° C]), decreased breath sounds and crackles on auscultation, worsening ABG levels, an increased A-a oxygen gradient, and decreased lung compliance. A chest X-ray confirms the presence of infiltrates.

You can help prevent atelectasis by setting the sigh mechanism to periodically increase tidal volume and by making sure the patient receives humidified gas. Suction and reposition him as needed, and perform chest physiotherapy. If mucus and secretions cause significant obstruction, the patient may need fiber-optic bronchoscopy.

Barotrauma. Mechanical ventilation can increase air pressure in the lungs, causing barotrauma—lung tissue damage from excessive air pressure. If prolonged, barotrauma can cause chronic lung function loss. In infants, such damage can cause bronchopulmonary dysplasia, a chronic obstructive disorder.

Barotrauma results from alveoli leaking gas into the extraparenchymal structures, trauma, chest tube insertion, a fractured rib, pulmonary tissue damage, ruptured blebs, a ruptured bronchus, or a newly inserted tracheostomy tube that lets air leak in around it.

Certain procedures and disorders increase the risk of barotrauma. These include surgery, closed chest compression, subclavian vein needle puncture, chest trauma, acute restrictive lung disease requiring PEEP higher than 10 cm H_2O, and severe, preexisting pulmonary disease, such as COPD. Other factors that heighten the risk of barotrauma include PEEP or CPAP therapy and ventilator settings that increase peak inspiratory pressure above 40 cm H_2O.

The three most common types of barotrauma are pneumothorax, tension pneumothorax, and pneumomediastinum.

• *Pneumothorax.* Air in the pleural space, or pneumothorax, causes lung tissue compression. The more air present in the pleural space, the more the lung tissue compresses, decreasing the number of alveoli available for gas exchange. This leads to hypoxemia.

The patient may show signs of respiratory distress, including dys-

Understanding atelectasis

These illustrations show normal lung tissue, the start of atelectasis, and complete alveolar collapse.

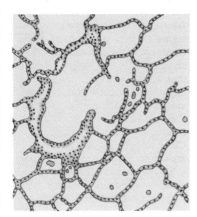

Normal lung tissue has clearly defined alveoli bounded by capillaries.

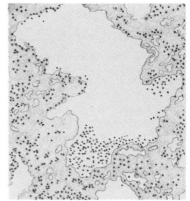

This close-up of an alveolus shows the initial inflammatory changes of parenchymal infection. Lung consolidation begins as fibrin and microemboli start forming in the alveoli, decreasing the number of functioning alveoli. Fibrin, blood, and cellular debris eventually fill the alveoli, resulting in pneumonia.

pnea, restlessness, cyanosis, vital sign changes, elevated peak inspiratory pressure, decreased breath sounds and chest movement on the affected side, subcutaneous emphysema, and chest X-ray changes, such as a shift in the trachea, mediastinum, or other structures and a loss of lung markings. If the pneumothorax is large, the doctor may aspirate the air from the pleural space, either with a needle or a chest tube.

To assess for pneumothorax, check for subcutaneous emphysema by palpating the skin at tube sites, the neck, and the upper chest. As you palpate, listen for a crackling or popping sound, a possible sign of pneumothorax.

• *Tension pneumothorax.* A buildup of air in the pleural space can result in a tension pneumothorax—a life-threatening disorder. The increased pressure in the pleural space can shift the mediastinum, great vessels, atria, and ventricles and collapse the lung, impeding ventilation and causing total circulatory collapse. The patient must receive chest decompression immediately to prevent death.

Monitor a patient with pneumothorax closely for signs of a tension

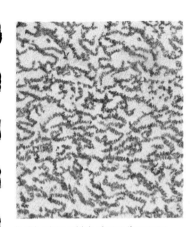

In this view, which shows the same area as the first illustration, complete alveolar collapse has occurred. Note that the clearly defined alveoli are now gone. Instead, you see consolidated lung tissue that impairs both ventilation and oxygenation.

pneumothorax. These include severe dyspnea and restlessness, cyanosis, a weak and rapid pulse, decreased blood pressure, a sudden increase in peak inspiratory pressure with a decrease in tidal volume, decreased PaO_2, increased A-a oxygen gradient, asymmetrical thoracic expansion, tracheal deviation, hyperresonance, and, ultimately, shock and cardiac arrest. If you detect such signs, notify the doctor immediately, and be prepared to assist with chest decompression.

• *Pneumomediastinum.* You can detect air in the mediastinum by auscultating a crunching or bubbling sound on inspiration that occurs in synchrony with the heartbeat. If the mediastinum traps too much air, the elevated pressure can compress the heart muscle and significantly decrease cardiac output.

Decreased venous return. The increased pressure that PEEP and CPAP generate expands alveoli, constricting the pulmonary vasculature that surrounds them. The pressure impedes blood flow and reduces the amount of blood that can enter the chest cavity, decreasing preload. Increasing the level of PEEP or CPAP aggravates the situation, ultimately reducing cardiac output.

You'll notice the effects of decreased cardiac output most in patients receiving high-level PEEP therapy and in those with CHF or in hypovolemic shock. Signs include an increased heart rate, decreased blood pressure, and a drop in urine output. Making sure the patient has a sufficient fluid volume may increase right ventricular preload. If that doesn't work, the patient may need an inotropic agent, such as dopamine or dobutamine, to increase cardiac contractility.

GI alterations. Mechanical ventilation puts stress on the entire body, and that causes gastric acid secretion and gastric irritation. The ventilator patient who is NPO may develop stress ulcers and GI bleeding. Patients who already have peptic ulcers or who are on long-term steroid or salicylate therapy run an even greater risk. The stomach wall starts to break down within 24 hours of the patient being NPO, so tube feedings should start right away for patients with functional GI tracts to reduce the risk of gastric irritation and stress ulcers. Antacids and histamine-2 receptor antagonists can help, too, by keeping the gastric pH at 3.5 or higher. Monitor the patient for ulcers and bleeding by testing his stomach aspirate and stools for blood.

Stress can also cause gastric distention and intestinal obstruction. Auscultate for bowel sounds every 4 hours. Hypoactive or absent bowel sounds may indicate a paralytic ileus. Check for residual food in the intestines from tube feeding before starting intermittent feedings, to monitor for gastric distention.

Infection. A patient's upper respiratory flora change less than 48 hours after mechanical ventilation begins. As long as the tracheal wall remains intact, the patient can withstand the colonization of this hospital-acquired flora. But as suctioning, tube placement, and cuff inflation alter the tracheal mucosa, the risk of infection increases.

Debilitation and immunosuppression increase the infection risk even further. And the equipment itself can be an assault on the patient. The airway tube stops him from coughing to clear upper air passages. Use of aerosols and unsterile or frequent suctioning can introduce more microbes. Central lines add more possible infection sites. And the patient may damage his pulmonary system by aspirating gastric contents.

You can help prevent cross-contamination by washing your hands thoroughly before treating the patient and by using aseptic technique and sterile equipment. Change the ventilator tubing every 24 to 48 hours, depending on hospital policy. Always use sterile technique for suctioning, and suction only as needed. Perform chest physiotherapy to help remove retained secretions, which can encourage

microbial growth. Monitor for signs of respiratory tract infection, particularly a temperature above 102° F (38.9° C) and a change in the amount or color of secretions. If an infection develops, obtain a specimen for culture and sensitivity testing.

Oxygen toxicity. When a patient receives oxygen at concentrations above 50%, he runs the risk of oxygen toxicity. Oxygen can cause fibrosis, edema, and thickening of the interstitial spaces, and can interfere with surfactant, causing capillary congestion.

You can help prevent oxygen toxicity by monitoring ABG levels. Adjust oxygen delivery so that the patient's PaO_2 remains at 60 mm Hg and his arterial oxygen saturation stays at 90%, while keeping FIO_2 as low as possible — preferably at or below 0.4. Maintain good pulmonary hygiene so you can keep the oxygen concentration low. Reduce a high oxygen concentration as soon as the patient can tolerate the reduction.

Watch the patient for signs and symptoms of oxygen toxicity. These include retrosternal distress, paresthesia in the extremities, nausea and vomiting, anorexia, fatigue, lethargy, malaise, dyspnea, coughing, and restlessness. Late signs include progressive respiratory difficulty, cyanosis, dyspnea, and asphyxia. Pulmonary changes include a decrease in compliance and vital capacity with an increase in the A-a oxygen gradient.

Psychological complications
Mechanical ventilation doesn't just affect the patient's body; it can have a profound psychological impact, too. Not only is the patient in an unfamiliar setting, but his body has

been invaded with tubes and catheters that stop him from moving freely, even from speaking. His feelings of not being in control can cause fear and anxiety, and, in turn, a stress response.

So be alert for signs and symptoms of such a response, including increased gastric secretions, dilated pupils, dry mouth, peripheral vasoconstriction, and increased heart rate, blood pressure, and respiratory rate. The stress response may decrease as the patient better understands the therapy and becomes more comfortable with it, but the accompanying sleep loss — particularly the loss of REM sleep — can still cause stress and fear. Also, the continuous stimuli of the hospital routine and the equipment mean little to the patient, so his mind may start to drift, leaving him unfocused.

You can reduce stress and keep the patient alert and interested by making sure he has a calendar and clock in sight to help keep him oriented. Make sure he has a way of communicating, and encourage family members to visit often. If possible, try to arrange for the same personnel to treat the patient, so he becomes familiar with them. Make sure he has at least 4 hours of uninterrupted sleep. And keep reassuring him and talking to him.

Discontinuing mechanical ventilation

The day a patient begins mechanical ventilation therapy, you should start planning for weaning — the gradual withdrawal of the patient from ventilator support. If you don't, the weaning process may take longer than necessary. As soon as mechanical ventilation begins, start measures to keep the patient's respiratory muscles conditioned. If his condition permits, use ventilation modes, such as IMV or ACV, that allow as much spontaneous breathing as possible. And begin weaning as soon as the patient is able.

Deciding when to wean

Usually, you can start to wean a patient when the underlying cause of respiratory insufficiency has been successfully treated. However, the patient must meet certain other criteria. He must be able to maintain adequate ventilation with spontaneous breathing. Plus, he must have a stable cardiovascular system, with intrapulmonary shunts of no more than 20% of total pulmonary blood flow. He should have sufficient respiratory muscle strength to maintain spontaneous breathing. And he must have a level of consciousness that will let him sustain breathing. (For other criteria, see *Weaning the patient from the ventilator,* page 170.)

Thoroughly assess the patient's physical and mental status before attempting to wean him from ventilator therapy. Pay particular attention to his cardiovascular status, nutritional status, and level of consciousness.

Cardiovascular status. Check the hemodynamic measurements that reflect the heart's ability to pump oxygenated blood. For successful weaning, the patient should have an adequate cardiac output and cardiac index. He should have a normal fluid balance (determined by measuring central pressures), an indication that his heart isn't overworking because of increased blood volume.

Weaning the patient from the ventilator

Successful weaning hinges on the patient's ability to breathe on his own. That means he must have a spontaneous respiratory effort that can keep him ventilated, a stable cardiovascular system, and sufficient respiratory muscle strength and level of consciousness to sustain spontaneous breathing. He also should meet some or all of the following criteria:

☐ Pao$_2$ of 60 mm Hg (50 mm Hg or the ability to maintain baseline levels if he has chronic lung disease) or an FIO$_2$ at or below 0.4

☐ Paco$_2$ of less than 40 mm Hg or normal for the patient, or an FIO$_2$ of 0.4 or less if his Paco$_2$ is 60 mm Hg or more

☐ A vital capacity of more than 10 ml/kg of body weight

☐ Maximum inspiratory pressure of more than -20 cm H$_2$O

☐ Minute ventilation of less than 10 liters/minute with a respiratory frequency of less than 24 breaths/minute

☐ FEV$_1$ of more than 10 ml/kg of body weight

☐ Ability to double his spontaneous resting minute ventilation

☐ Adequate natural airway or a functioning tracheostomy

☐ Ability to cough effectively enough to mobilize secretions

☐ Ability to breathe without pancuronium or other neuromuscular blocker or sedation

☐ Clear or clearing chest X-ray

☐ Absence of infection, acid-base or electrolyte imbalance, hyperglycemia, arrhythmias, renal failure, anemia, fever, or excessive fatigue.

A normal hemoglobin level means his blood has normal viscosity and can carry sufficient oxygen. And a normal potassium level will help prevent arrhythmias and maintain normal myocardial contractility.

Nutritional status. Make sure the patient receives enough nutrition to maintain respiratory muscles. Check the results of metabolic studies to ensure that he doesn't take in more carbohydrates than he needs. Metabolizing carbohydrates increases CO$_2$ production, which, in turn, increases the work of breathing needed to release the CO$_2$. And the increased work of breathing means respiratory muscles need more oxygen. Without oxygen, the respiratory muscles can grow fatigued and hinder weaning.

Level of consciousness. To be weaned successfully, the patient must maintain a level of consciousness that at least allows spontaneous respirations to occur. Ideally, he'll be awake, alert, and oriented. You'll have a better idea of what level of consciousness the patient should reach before you start weaning by knowing his prognosis and what his level of consciousness was before ventilation began. Check the extent and location of any tissue damage, and make sure he is properly oxygenated, has a stable cardiovascular status, and gets enough sleep — all factors that affect level of consciousness.

Weaning method
The selection of a weaning method depends on whether the patient originally needed mechanical ventilation to correct oxygenation failure or ventilatory failure.

Oxygenation failure. If the patient needed mechanical ventilation for oxygenation, he must be able to tolerate decreased levels of PEEP and a lower FIO$_2$. Decrease his PEEP

Comparing weaning methods

You can use one of several methods to wean a patient from mechanical ventilation. These include the intermittent mandatory ventilation (IMV), synchronized intermittent mandatory ventilation (SIMV), assist-control ventilation (ACV), T-piece, and pressure-support ventilation (PSV) methods.

METHOD	CHARACTERISTICS	INDICATIONS
IMV or SIMV	• Gradually increases the interval between ventilator-delivered breaths until all ventilations are spontaneous • At lower settings, allows more even air dispersal in the lungs • Helps prevent muscle atrophy and incoordination	• Elderly or debilitated patients • Patients with chronic pulmonary or muscular disorders • Patients who are difficult to wean • Patients who fear being off the ventilator
ACV	• Allows patient to initiate mechanically supported breaths • Allows progression from continuous ventilator support to intervals during which the patient breaths through a T-piece	• Patients on prolonged continuous mandatory ventilation • Patients who are difficult to wean • Patients who need respiratory muscle reconditioning
T-piece (conventional)	• Allows delivery of oxygen and humidity • Allows periodic removal from the ventilator until spontaneous breathing resumes	• Patients who've been on ventilator therapy less than 2 days • Long-term ventilator patients who are not psychologically dependent on the ventilator
PSV	• Augments the patient's spontaneous breaths with positive pressure • Gradually decreases level of pressure	• Long-term ventilator patients with muscular atrophy who are psychologically dependent on the ventilator

in increments of 3 to 5 cm H_2O, making sure to maintain a PaO_2 of at least 60 mm Hg and an FIO_2 of 0.4 or less. Adjust the ventilator rate, mode, and volume to keep pH between 7.35 and 7.45. You'll know you've weaned the patient when the PEEP level reaches or drops below 5 cm H_2O with an FIO_2 of 0.4. The doctor will extubate him after he's been on CPAP successfully for 2 to 6 hours.

Ventilatory failure. For a patient who has suffered ventilatory failure, the doctor will choose from among several weaning methods, including IMV or SIMV, ACV, T-piece (sometimes used with CPAP), or PSV. (See *Comparing weaning methods*.) The IMV, SIMV, or ACV methods (commonly used alternately with CPAP) can initially help patients who are difficult to wean — elderly, debilitated patients with chronic pulmonary or neuromuscular disease, for instance.

• *IMV or SIMV.* When you use IMV or SIMV to wean, decrease the number of ventilator-delivered breaths until the patient can breathe on his own. With either method, the patient will receive ventilatory support while his respiratory muscles build up endurance and become reconditioned. Plus, because these methods decrease the number of ventilator-delivered breaths gradually, they help ease the patient's fears of being off the ventilator.

IMV and SIMV do have some drawbacks, though. Because they require the patient to breathe completely on his own between ventilator-delivered breaths, they cause respiratory muscle fatigue. They also increase the risk of hypercapnia and cardiac decompensation in patients with underlying heart disease. And if you don't change the rate frequently enough, weaning will take longer than it should.

• *ACV*. Use this method to wean a patient from prolonged CMV. ACV helps recondition respiratory muscles by letting the patient initiate mechanically supported breaths. Weaning can continue with IMV and finally the T-piece method.

If the patient moves straight from ACV to the T-piece method, let him breathe humidified, oxygenated gas delivered through the T-piece for short periods of time each hour during the daytime without the support of the ventilator. Then gradually increase the amount of time the patient uses the T-piece. Start increasing it by 5 minutes each time until you've reached an hour, then by 15 minutes until you've reached 2 hours, then by 30 minutes until you've reached 4 hours. Keep the patient off the ventilator for 4 hours at a time, followed by 1 hour on the machine.

After that, increase nighttime weaning by an hour at a time until the patient only needs mechanical ventilation for 1-hour periods between 4-hour periods of breathing on his own. (Total ventilatory support at night during the first phase of weaning lets the patient's respiratory muscle function build up gradually.)

• *T-piece*. Use the T-piece method for patients who've been on the ventilator less than 2 days, including patients who have recently had cardiothoracic surgery, are in a drug-induced coma, or suffer from status asthmaticus or brief exacerbations of chronic lung disease. Give the patient oxygen through a T-piece once he wakes up. Measure ABG levels after 20 to 30 minutes and again after 1 to 4 hours. When the patient can maintain normal ABG levels, the doctor will extubate him.

You can also use the T-piece method for a patient on long-term therapy following the steps for using a T-piece with ACV. The spontaneously breathing patient may need CPAP, too, so his airways don't close up and cause atelectasis.

• *PSV*. To wean a patient with PSV, gradually decrease the level of pressure support until he can breathe on his own. You can combine PSV with SIMV.

Nursing considerations

No matter which weaning method you use on the patient, you'll follow some of the same basic steps to prepare him, monitor his response, and prevent any problems. Depending on the patient's condition, you may need to help him overcome physical or psychological barriers to weaning.

Explain the proposed plan to the patient and his family. Then place the patient in an upright position. If you seat the patient in a chair, wait 5 minutes after you've seated him to begin weaning. That way, he won't be too tired from the effort of sitting to begin weaning.

Take his vital signs and obtain an

ECG rhythm strip to use as baselines. During the weaning process, frequently assess the patient's vital signs and ventilatory parameters.

If you're using a T-piece, keep the ventilator close by in case the patient becomes too tired and needs ventilator support sooner than planned. If you're using IMV, be ready to start machine-delivered breaths, either when the patient has successfully breathed on his own for the specified period of time or when it's clear that he can't yet tolerate spontaneous breathing. And no matter which method you're using, stay with the patient to reassure and calm him.

Barriers to weaning. Long-term mechanical ventilation can render a patient psychologically and physically dependent on the ventilator. Monitor his mental and emotional state, and frequently assess his psychological adaptation to weaning. Encourage him to persist with weaning, but reassure him that you can return him to the ventilator if necessary.

Stop the weaning process and return the patient to the ventilator if you observe physical indications that he isn't ready to be weaned. These indications include arrhythmias, increased work of breathing, or a significantly increased blood pressure, heart rate, or respiratory rate. (For a more complete list of physical signs, see *When to stop weaning*.)

Weaning may fail if the patient can't meet his ventilatory requirement or if he has hypoxemia, respiratory muscle fatigue (from an unresolved underlying lung disease), or decreased cardiac output. Excessive secretions, a weak cough, impaired mucociliary clearing, and ineffective suctioning also under-

When to stop weaning

Discontinue weaning and return the patient to the ventilator if you detect any of these signs:
- ☐ Blood pressure rise of more than 20 mm Hg systolic or more than 10 mm Hg diastolic
- ☐ Heart rate increase of more than 20 beats/minute or a rate above 120 beats/minute
- ☐ Respiratory rate increase of more than 10 breaths/minute or a rate above 30 breaths/minute
- ☐ Arrhythmias
- ☐ Reduced tidal volume
- ☐ Elevated $PaCO_2$
- ☐ Anxiety
- ☐ Dyspnea
- ☐ Accessory muscle use or deteriorating breathing pattern

mine weaning. The underlying problems should be resolved before attempting to wean the patient.

Monitoring the patient. To determine when the patient is completely weaned, you'll need to monitor his vital capacity, negative inspiratory force, forced expiratory volume in 1 second (FEV_1), minute ventilation, maximal minute ventilation, shunt, A-a oxygen gradient, and Vd/Vt. Note when these measurements return to normal. When you move the patient from partial ventilatory support to a T-piece or CPAP, make sure that his PaO_2 doesn't change and that his $PaCO_2$ changes no more than 5 mm Hg — two of the most frequently used indicators of successful weaning.

For a patient with chronic lung disease, the $PaCO_2$ may return to its preventilator level. Also, weaning may take longer — anywhere from several days to weeks. This allows the kidneys time to increase production of bicarbonate to buffer the additional hydrogen ions that accompany the increased CO_2 levels associated with chronic lung disease. Otherwise, the patient's pH could drop below 7.35.

Extubation

The doctor can remove the artificial airway when the patient no longer needs mechanical ventilation. Extubation of orally or nasally inserted tubes decreases airway resistance and the work of breathing.

If the patient has a tracheostomy tube, the doctor may delay extubation for a while after the patient has been successfully weaned. Otherwise, the patient will need the tube surgically reinserted if a ventilatory problem develops. While the patient waits for extubation, he may have a fenestrated tube — a tube with holes through the outer cannula — inserted, or his tracheostomy tube may be closed off with a trach button. If he needs mechanical ventilation again, he can have an inner cannula inserted that will occlude the fenestrations or have the trach button removed. If the fenestrated tube interferes with airflow, maintain the tracheostomy with a stent.

Assisting with extubation. To prepare for extubation, gather the following equipment: manual resuscitation bag with a mask and 1.0 FIO_2, a 10-cc non-luer-lock syringe, intubation equipment, and a high-humidity oxygen delivery system. Explain the procedure to the patient. Then elevate his head and check his vital signs. Set up the oxygen delivery system to use after extubation, and have the manual resuscitation bag and intubation equipment ready.

Suction the patient's upper airway and oropharynx before the doctor extubates him. Deflate the cuff with the syringe. The doctor will remove the tube when the patient has finished taking a breath with the manual resuscitation bag. To ease extubation, have the patient cough while the doctor removes the tube.

Follow-up care. After the patient has been extubated, place him on a high-humidity oxygen delivery system to help prevent laryngospasm. Check his vital signs, and recheck them and his ABG levels 20 minutes after extubation. Monitor him for signs of laryngospasm — inspiratory stridor and dyspnea. Watch for complications, including acute laryngeal edema, hoarseness, and aspiration. The patient may also develop later complications, including fibrotic stenosis of the trachea, tracheoesophageal fistula, and laryngeal stenosis. If later complications develop, the doctor will need to dilate the patient's airway, surgically open the airway, or insert a permanent tracheostomy tube.

Suggested readings

Cardiopulmonary Emergencies. Springhouse, Pa.: Springhouse Corp., 1991.

Difillipo, N.M., and Jenkins, A.J. "Pressure Support Ventilation," *American Family Physician* 38(2):147-50, August 1988.

Kinney, M.R., et al. *AACN'S Clinical Reference for Critical-Care Nursing,* 2nd ed. New York: McGraw-Hill Book Co., 1988.

Lain, D.C., et al. "Pressure Control Inverse Ratio Ventilation as a Method to Reduce Peak Inspiratory Pressure and Provide Adequate Ventilation and Oxygenation," *Chest* 95(5):1081-88, May 1989.

MacIntyre, N.R. "New Forms of Mechanical Ventilation in the Adult," *Clinical Chest Medicine* 9(1):47-54, March 1988.

MacIntyre, N.R. "Pressure Support Ventilation: Effects on Ventilatory Reflexes and Ventilatory-Muscle Workloads," *Respiratory Care* 32(6):447-57, June 1987.

Norton, L.C., and Neureuter, A. "Weaning the Long-Term Ventilator-dependent Patient: Common Problems and Management," *Critical Care Nurse* 9(1):42-52, January 1989.

Slutsky, A.S. "Nonconventional Methods of Ventilation," *American Review of Respiratory Disease* 138(1):175-83, July 1988.

Stock, M.C., et al. "Airway Pressure Release Ventilation," *Critical Care Medicine* 15(5):462-66, May 1987.

Tharratt R.S., et al. "Pressure Controlled Inverse Ratio Ventilation in Severe Adult Respiratory Failure," *Chest* 94(4):755-62, October 1988.

Vasbinder-Dillon, D. "Understanding Mechanical Ventilation," *Critical Care Nurse* 8(7):42-43, October 1988.

6

CHEST DRAINAGE

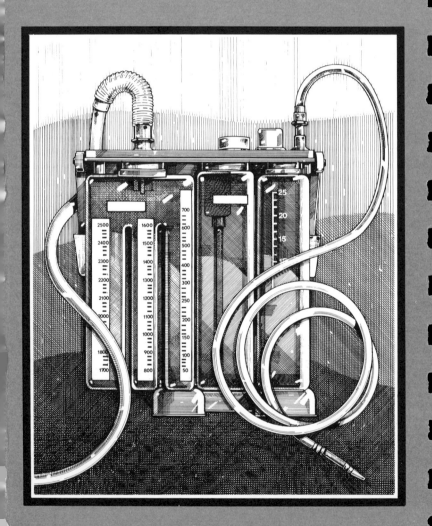

Normally, negative pressure in the pleural space keeps the lungs from collapsing. But air or fluid leaking into that space can disrupt this negative pressure, leading to a partial or complete lung collapse—a potentially life-threatening condition.

To drain such accumulated air or fluid, a doctor will insert a chest tube into the pleural space. This tube, which is connected to a chest drainage system, restores normal intrapleural pressure, so the patient can maintain normal cardiopulmonary function.

Although a doctor will actually insert the chest tube, you'll need to be familiar with the procedure and its indications. This chapter will tell you how to assist with chest tube insertion, care for the patient, and monitor the drainage system. The chapter also explains how to recognize complications and intervene appropriately. Finally, the chapter discusses when and how to discontinue chest drainage therapy.

Basics of chest drainage

To understand how chest tubes and drainage systems work, you need to review normal breathing first. Breathing operates on the principle that gases move from an area of greater pressure to one of lower pressure. (See *Understanding terms used in chest drainage.*) *Intrapulmonic pressure,* or the pressure in the lungs, normally fluctuates between subatmospheric (negative) pressure and just slightly above atmospheric pressure. This fluctuation causes the air to move in and out of the lungs. *Intrapleural pressure,* or the pressure between the

Understanding terms used in chest drainage

Review the following terms to gain a clearer understanding of chest drainage.

Atmospheric pressure. The normal pressure exerted by the atmosphere—760 mm Hg at sea level.

Negative pressure. A pressure less than atmospheric pressure. It exerts a pulling force.

Positive pressure. A pressure greater than atmospheric pressure. It exerts a pushing force.

Parietal pleura. The thin membrane that lines the chest cavity.

Visceral pleura. The thin membrane that lines the lungs.

Pleural cavity. The potential space between the visceral and the parietal pleurae.

Chylothorax. An accumulation of chyle in the pleural cavity from the thoracic duct.

Hemopneumothorax. An accumulation of both air and blood or serosanguineous fluid in the pleural cavity.

Hemothorax. An accumulation of bloody fluid in the pleural cavity.

Pleural effusion. An accumulation of fluid in the pleural cavity, possibly from a malignant tumor.

Pneumothorax. An accumulation of air in the pleural cavity.

Pyothorax. An accumulation of pus in the pleural cavity. Also called empyema.

parietal and visceral pleurae, is always negative. This negative pressure prevents the lungs from collapsing even though the elasticity of the lung tissue makes them want to recoil. When a patient loses negative intrapleural pressure, lung tissue collapses and the alveoli in that lung area become unavailable for gas exchange. Intrapleural collections of blood, serous fluid, chyle, and pus also cause lung tissue to collapse.

A chest tube and drainage system can remove excess fluid as well as air. In an emergency, you may insert a flutter valve.

Indications

A doctor may insert a chest tube for an open, closed, or tension pneumothorax. It's also indicated for hemothorax, pyothorax, pleural effusion, or chylothorax.

In an *open pneumothorax,* air usually enters the pleural space through a surgical incision or a traumatic chest wound. The opening in the chest wall allows atmospheric air (atmospheric pressure) to flow directly into the pleural cavity (negative pressure). As the pressure becomes more positive, the lung collapses on the affected side.

In a *closed pneumothorax,* air enters the pleural space through the lung, increasing pleural pressure and preventing lung expansion during normal inspiration.

A potentially fatal condition, *tension pneumothorax* requires immediate intervention. It occurs when air enters the pleural space either from within the lung, as with lung or airway damage, or from outside the lung, as with a sucking chest wound that creates a one-way valve effect. Air enters the pleural space, but without a chest tube, it can't escape. The accumulating pressure

causes partial or total lung collapse, usually with mediastinal shift. The heart, trachea, esophagus, and great vessels are pushed to the unaffected side, compressing the heart and the contralateral lung and significantly decreasing cardiac output.

Chest tubes

Also called a thoracotomy tube or a thoracic catheter, a chest tube is a firm plastic drain with several eyelets in the proximal end. The number of chest tubes used and their insertion sites depend on two factors: the patient's injury and the type of material being drained.

Gravity naturally causes heavier material, such as fluids, to accumulate in the bottom of the cavity, and lighter material, such as air, to accumulate at the top. If only air has accumulated — as in pneumothorax — the doctor will usually insert the chest tube in the anterior chest at the midclavicular line in the second or third intercostal space. If fluid, such as blood, chyle, or pus, has accumulated, the doctor will insert the chest tube lower, at the midaxillary line in the fourth to sixth intercostal space.

Chest drainage systems

Closed chest drainage systems attach to a chest tube to collect excess air and fluid. They come in two basic types: bottle and disposable. (See *Comparing closed drainage systems.*) Bottle systems use one, two, or three bottles to collect drainage, create a water seal, and control suction. Disposable systems combine the features of a multibottle system in a compact, one-piece unit. Although you're less likely to use the bottle system, its principles form the foundation for your understanding of how the disposable system works.

EQUIPMENT

Comparing closed drainage systems

One-bottle system

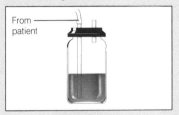

From patient

- Easiest system to use
- Drains by gravity
- Combines drainage collection and water-seal chamber
- Not recommended for excessive drainage

Two-bottle system

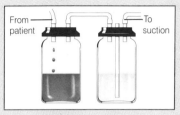

From patient — To suction

- Separates functions: first bottle serves as drainage collection chamber; second bottle acts as the water-seal chamber
- Not recommended for excessive drainage

Three-bottle system

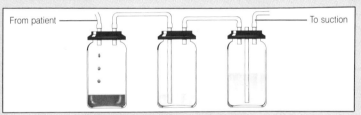

From patient — To suction

- Separates functions: first bottle serves as drainage collection chamber; second bottle as the water-seal chamber; third bottle as the suction-control chamber
- Adequately handles excessive drainage

Disposable system

- Combines drainage collection, water-seal, and suction-control chambers in one unit
- Ensures patient safety with one-way seal
- Easily visible air-leak indicator
- Pressure indicator confirms working order
- Automatically protects the patient with positive and negative pressure relief valves
- Quiet; no bubbling sound

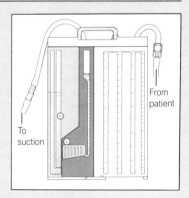

To suction

From patient

One-bottle system. This system consists of one bottle that serves as both a drainage collection chamber and a water-seal chamber. The distal end of the chest tube connects to the latex drainage tubing, which connects to a rigid straw. The straw extends into the single sterile glass or plastic bottle, resting about 1″ (2.5 cm) below the water level, creating a water seal that prevents atmospheric air from entering the tubing and the pleura. During inspiration and expiration, pleural air escapes through the tubing into the water and out the vent in the top of the bottle. The water acts as a one-way valve, allowing pleural air out but preventing atmospheric air from entering.

Expect the water level to fluctuate as the patient breathes; the level goes up when he inhales and down when he exhales. You also may detect air bubbles at the end of the drainage tubing.

Two-bottle system. With a two-bottle system, the drainage collection chamber is separate from the water-seal chamber. The drainage collects in the first bottle, and the air flows through it into the second bottle, which serves as the water-seal chamber. The first bottle keeps the negative pressure at a fixed level and lets you more accurately observe the volume and type of drainage.

As with the one-bottle system, a vent in the second bottle allows incoming pleural air to escape. Bubbling from an air leak and fluctuations in the water level also may occur.

Three-bottle system. This system contains a drainage collection chamber, a water-seal chamber, and a suction-control chamber. The addi-

tion of the suction-control chamber is the safest way to regulate the amount of suction so that excessive negative pressure isn't exerted within the chest.

The depth of the venting tube in water controls the amount of suction, and the depth of the straw in water determines the maximum level of suction that can be exerted. The tube is submerged to a depth that exerts a pressure ranging from -10 to -20 cm H_2O (the normal negative pressure in the chest). No matter what the source of the negative pressure, the suction reaching the patient will be no greater than the pressure exerted by the length of the submerged tube.

Suction is applied to the pleura until negative pressure equals the positive pressure as generated by the water level. If the suction is turned higher, it will only increase the bubbling in the control bottle, not the amount of suction.

Disposable drainage systems. Of the two disposable drainage systems available, the water-seal type is used more commonly than the newer waterless type.

Examples of the compact water-seal units include the Atrium Compact, ConMed Pleura-Gard, Deknatel Pleur-evac, Emerson 550, and Sherwood Medical Thora-seal systems. Most of these units have an optional removable fourth container that attaches to the unit for autotransfusion. (See *Using autotransfusion for chest wounds.*)

Water-seal systems work similar to the three-bottle system. The first compartment collects the fluid drained from the chest; the second compartment, the water-seal chamber, allows pleural air to escape but prevents the return of atmo-

Using autotransfusion for chest wounds

Autotransfusion consists of collecting, filtering, and reinfusing a patient's own blood. Most often used for chest wounds, it can also be used whenever two or three units of pooled blood can be recovered, as in heart or orthopedic surgery. Because it uses the patient's own blood, autotransfusion eliminates the risk of transfusion reactions and transmitting cytomegalovirus, hepatitis, acquired immunodeficiency syndrome, and other blood-borne diseases. It is contraindicated in patients with cancer or sepsis.

How autotransfusion works

First, the blood is collected from a wound or body cavity, using a large-bore chest tube connected to a closed drainage system. This blood passes through a filter into a collection bag. This filter catches most potential thrombi, such as clumps of fibrin and

damaged red blood cells. From the bag, the blood can be reinfused immediately or processed in a commercial cell washer that reduces anticoagulated whole blood to washed red blood cells for later infusion.

How to assist with autotransfusion

- To prepare for an autotransfusion, set up the collection system as you would any closed chest drainage system. Then attach the autotransfusion collection bag according to the manufacturer's instructions.
- If ordered, inject an anticoagulant into the self-sealing port on the connector of the patient's drainage tubing.
- During reinfusion, monitor the patient for complications, such as blood clotting, hemolysis, coagulopathies, thrombocytopenia, particulate and air emboli, sepsis, and citrate toxicity.

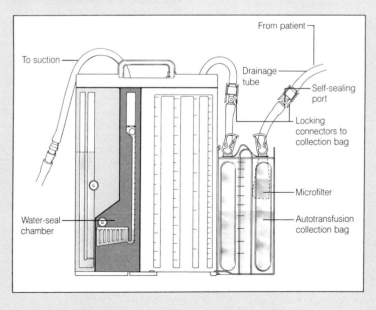

spheric air; and the third compartment controls suction. The amount of water in the third chamber determines the degree of suction.

The waterless systems have several advantages over the water-seal systems. They have one less chamber to fill, present no evaporation problems, and operate more quietly. These systems, which include the Argyle-Sentinel Seal and Davol Thora-Klex, use a mechanical screw-type valve to regulate suction. This valve replaces the traditional water column in a suction-control bottle. The screw valve works by varying the size of the opening to the suction pump. Because the valve is narrow at any setting, these drainage systems can suction only limited volumes of air.

Another waterless system, Pleurevac A-6000, uses a carefully calibrated spring mechanism to regulate the suction. By turning a dial on the side of the control chamber, you place a precise amount of tension on a spring in the top part of the chamber, which is open to the atmosphere. The spring pulls on a rubber seal that closes off an opening to the bottom part of the chamber and prevents atmospheric air from reentering. The higher the suction setting, the more tension on the spring and the more firmly the opening closes. The suction apparatus connects to the bottom part of the chamber via an internal channel. When the desired level of suction is reached, the negative pressure in the bottom part of the chamber is high enough to pull the rubber seal off the spring. This allows air to enter from the top part of the chamber and offsets any further suction.

Flutter valve

The flutter valve allows accumulated air and fluid to escape during expiration without admitting air during inspiration. The valve has a length of tubing flattened at one end and is encased by a plastic cylinder that protects it from external compression and occlusion. Should the cylinder crack or break, the flutter valve would still work.

A flutter valve is indicated for a patient with a small, slowly resolving pneumothorax or a patient being transferred to another floor. It may also be temporarily attached to a needle after an emergency needle thoracotomy, remaining in place only until the patient can be connected to a chest tube and a drainage system. (See *Performing needle thoracotomy*.) A sterile glove or dressing can be placed on the distal end of the valve to collect drainage. The drainage collection device must be vented so that air exiting the chest will not be trapped.

Initiating and maintaining chest drainage

When a doctor inserts a chest tube, you may have to assist. Once it's in place, you'll routinely assess the patient and note any complications. You'll also need to check the chest drainage system frequently to make sure it's working properly.

Assisting with chest tube insertion

Before chest tube insertion, the doctor will have the patient sign an informed consent form. You should make sure the patient understands why he needs a chest tube and what the procedure entails.

To assist with the insertion, collect a chest tube tray with the

Performing needle thoracotomy

For a patient with life-threatening tension pneumothorax, a needle thoracotomy temporarily relieves pleural pressure until a doctor can insert a chest tube.

How needle thoracotomy works

A needle, attached to a flutter valve, is inserted into the affected pleural space. (If no flutter valve is available, one can be made from a perforated finger cot or glove and attached with a rubber band.) Trapped air escapes via the flutter valve when the patient exhales, instead of being retained under pressure. The flutter valve also prevents more air from entering the patient's lung during inhalation.

How to perform the procedure

If a doctor isn't available, you may need to perform this procedure.

Here's how to proceed:

• Clean the skin around the second intercostal space at the midclavicular line, using povidone-iodine solution. Use a circular motion, starting at the center and working outward.

• Insert a sterile 16G or larger needle over the superior portion of the rib and through the tissue covering the pleural cavity. The vein, artery, and nerve sit behind the rib's inferior border.

• Listen for a hissing sound. This signals the needle's entry into the pleural cavity.

• If you're using a flutter valve, secure it to the needle. The arrow on the valve indicates the direction of airflow.

• Place a sterile glove on the distal end of the valve to collect the drainage.

• Leave the needle in place until a chest tube can be inserted.

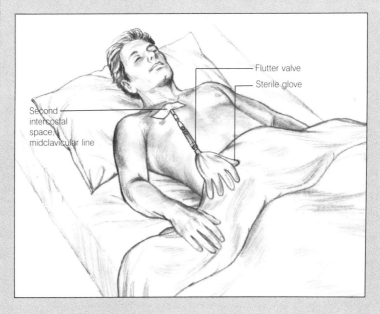

following equipment: sterile drape, alcohol swab, scalpel (usually with #11 blade), sterile forceps, two rubber-tipped clamps for each chest tube inserted, sterile 4″ × 4″ gauze sponges, two sterile 4″ × 4″ drain sponges (gauze sponges with slit), chest tube with trocar, sterile suture material (usually 20 silk with cutting needle), safety pin, and sterile drainage tubing (about 6′ long) and connector. Also collect two sets of sterile gloves, povidone-iodine solution, vial of 1% lidocaine, 10-ml syringe, 22G 1″ and 25G ⅝″ needles, 3″ or 4″ adhesive tape (or nonallergenic tape if the patient is allergic to adhesive tape), and the chest drainage system. If the doctor will be inserting two chest tubes on the same side, also obtain a Y-connector.

Then follow these steps:

• Using the manufacturer's instructions, prepare the chest drainage system so it can be connected to the chest tube after insertion.

• Position the patient appropriately, based on the intended insertion site (see *Positioning the patient for chest tube insertion*).

• Give the patient the ordered sedative. Then obtain the local anesthetic that the doctor will give just before the insertion. Warn the patient to expect considerable pressure during the insertion, but explain that the discomfort will last only a short time.

• Place the chest tube tray on the overbed table and open it, maintaining the sterile field. The doctor will put on sterile gloves, prepare the skin around the insertion site by cleaning it with povidone-iodine solution, and drape the patient.

• Wipe the rubber stopper of the anesthetic bottle with the alcohol swab. Then invert the bottle and hold it for the doctor to withdraw the anesthetic. After the doctor anesthetizes the site, he'll make a small incision and insert the chest tube. Then he'll either immediately connect the chest tube to the closed drainage unit or momentarily clamp the tube close to the patient's chest until he can connect it to the drainage system. After insertion, he may suture the tube to help prevent displacement.

• Next, open the packages containing the 4″ × 4″ drain sponges and gauze sponges, and put on sterile gloves. Place the drain sponges around the insertion site, one from above the tube and the other from below it. Then place several gauze sponges on top of the drain sponges. Tape the dressings, covering them completely.

• Tape the chest tube to the patient's chest distal to the insertion site to help prevent accidental tube dislodgment.

• Tape the junction of the chest tube and the drainage tubing to prevent separation.

• Coil the drainage tubing and secure it to the bed linen with tape and a safety pin, providing enough slack for the patient to move and turn. These measures help prevent the drainage tubing from dislodging, kinking, or dropping to the floor.

• Immediately after the drainage system is connected, tell the patient to take a deep breath. Have him hold it momentarily and then slowly exhale to help drain the pleural space and reexpand the lungs.

• Arrange for a portable chest X-ray to be taken to check the tube position.

Positioning the patient

After the tube is in place, position the patient properly and encourage him to cough and exhale to facilitate air and fluid drainage. Have him

site with a booted Kelly clamp. Have the patient take several breaths while you observe the water-seal chamber for bubbling. If no bubbles occur, the source of the leak is above the clamp — either at the insertion site or inside the patient. If bubbling continues after you clamp the chest tube, the air leak is in the drainage system below the clamp. Move the Kelly clamp about 4″ to 6″ (10 to 15 cm) down the tubing and check the water-seal chamber for bubbling again. Continue to move the clamp down the tubing in 4″ to 6″ increments and check for bubbling.

When the bubbling in the water-seal chamber stops, the leak is between the clamp's present position and its previous position. Try to seal the leak in the tube with tape. If the bubbling continues after you have moved the clamp down the entire length of the tube, the leak is in the drainage system itself and the system must be replaced.

Connections. If you haven't already done so, check the connections between the chest tube and the drainage tubing — as well as between the suction tubing and short latex tubing. The connections should be tight and wrapped with adhesive tape.

Dressing. Next, check the dressing to see that it's airtight, clean, dry, intact, and covered with adhesive tape. Don't remove the dressing unless you suspect the chest tube has moved or fluid is leaking around the insertion site, as indicated by drainage on the dressing. If you suspect a leak underneath the dressing, or if you have reason to believe that the insertion site is infected, remove the dressing and assess further.

Drainage. Now, assess the drainage, noting its amount, color, and consistency. Check drainage hourly for the first 24 hours after chest tube insertion, and then once every 2 hours. Make sure you know what material and how much of it should be draining. If you see anything unexpected, you know the patient has a problem and requires immediate attention. If the patient is actively bleeding, assess the drainage at least hourly. At no time should bloody drainage exceed 100 ml/ hour. If you find only a small amount (5 to 10 ml) of straw-colored drainage per shift, you need to measure the drainage only every 8 hours.

Correcting equipment problems

When you detect certain problems, you may be able to intervene to keep the drainage system functioning properly. (See *Managing problems of chest drainage,* page 188.) If you can't correct a malfunction quickly, you may need to assist the doctor with a needle thoracotomy or the insertion of another chest tube.

Loops in the drainage tubing. Dependent loops in the drainage tubing can impair therapy. To avoid this problem, coil the tubing flat on the bed and then let the remainder fall in a straight line to the drainage system. Next, secure the tubing to the bed by applying tape to the tubing and pinning the tape to the bed. Or try running the drainage tubing through a trough made in the bed linens. Create the trough by pinning two points of the bed sheet together and encasing the tubing in the fold (trough).

Keep in mind that sometimes, despite the best interventions, loops may form in the tubing. So you

Managing problems of chest drainage

PROBLEM	NURSING INTERVENTIONS
Patient rolls over on drainage tubing, causing obstruction.	• Reposition patient and remove any kinks in tubing. • Auscultate for decreased breath sounds and percuss for dullness, indicating fluid accumulation, or for hyperresonance, indicating air accumulation.
Dependent loops in tubing trap fluids and prevent effective drainage.	• Make sure chest drainage unit sits below patient's chest level. If necessary, raise the bed slightly to increase gravity flow. Remove kinks in tubing. • Monitor for decreased breath sounds and percuss for dullness.
No drainage appears in the collection chamber.	• If draining blood or other fluid, suspect a clot or obstruction in the tubing. Gently milk the tubing to expel the obstruction, if hospital policy permits. • Monitor the patient for lung tissue compression caused by accumulated pleural fluid.
Substantial increase in bloody drainage, indicating possible active bleeding or drainage of old blood.	• Monitor patient's vital signs. Look for increased pulse rate, decreased blood pressure, and orthostatic changes that may indicate acute blood loss. • Measure drainage every 15 to 30 minutes to determine if it's occurring continuously or in one gush caused by position changes.
No bubbling in the suction-control chamber.	• Check for obstructions in the tubing. Make sure connections are tight. • Check that suction apparatus is turned on. Increase suction slowly until you see gentle bubbling.
Loud, vigorous bubbling in the suction-control chamber	• Turn down the suction source until bubbling is just visible.
Evaporation causes the water level in the suction-control chamber to drop below desired − 20 cm H$_2$O.	• Using a syringe and needle, add water or saline solution through resealable diaphragm on back of suction-control chamber.
Patient has trouble breathing immediately after a special procedure. The chest drainage unit is improperly placed on his bed, interfering with drainage.	• Raise the head of the bed and reposition the unit so gravity promotes drainage. • Perform a quick respiratory assessment and take his vital signs. Check to ensure that there's enough water in the water-seal and suction-control chambers.
As the bed lowers, the chest drainage unit gets caught under the bed; the tubing comes apart and becomes contaminated.	• Clamp the chest tube proximal to the latex connection tubing. • Irrigate the tubing, using the sealed jar of sterile water or saline solution kept at the patient's bedside. • Insert the distal end of the chest tube into the jar of fluid until the end is 2 to 4 cm below the top of the water. Unclamp the chest tube. • Have another nurse obtain a new closed chest drainage system and set it up. • Attach the chest tube to the new unit.

need to observe and straighten the tubing frequently to help prevent problems.

Tubing obstructions. Another problem you may encounter is an obstruction in the tubing. Depending on your hospital's policy and procedure, you may be able to correct this problem by stripping (or milking) the tubing. This controversial technique creates a great deal of suction in a section of tubing. The result: Any clots or fibrin in the tubing are mechanically dislodged and pushed forward. Unfortunately, the suction may also cause the patient discomfort and cause tissue damage, such as bruising or entrapment.

The longer the section of tubing you compress, the more suction you create. This transient suction may exceed more than -100 cm H_2O when as little as 4" (10 cm) of tubing is stripped. It averages almost -300 cm H_2O when 18" (45 cm) is stripped and commonly exceeds -400 cm H_2O when the entire length is stripped.

Because the increase in suction creates excessive pressure in the pleura, stripping is no longer routinely performed. However, it may be indicated when a clot blocks the tubing — usually when fresh bleeding occurs. Stripping isn't necessary for a patient who has had heart surgery and has a mediastinal sump tube; the continuous flow of air through the pump's vent keeps it patent.

If stripping appears to be necessary, try this first: Squeeze the drainage tubing with a hand-over-hand motion. Release the tubing between each squeeze, or fan-fold several sections of tubing and then squeeze them. This technique is gentler than stripping and may be sufficient to dislodge the obstruction.

If your hospital's policy allows, strip the tubing by following these steps:
• Use an alcohol swab or hand lotion as a lubricant on the tubing to make the stripping easier.
• Grip and stabilize the tubing with the thumb and forefinger of one hand. Slide the thumb and forefinger of the other hand along the tubing from that point toward the collection chamber, compressing a section of the tubing.
• Then release the first hand and regrip the tubing where you've stopped, repeating the procedure along the entire length of the tubing.

Discontinuing therapy

Because prolonged intubation promotes infection, the doctor usually removes the chest tube within 5 to 7 days. Before removal, observe for these indications that the patient no longer needs the tube:
• Drainage diminishes to little or nothing.
• The air leak has disappeared.
• Fluctuations stop in the water-seal chamber.
• Solution creeps partway up the collection chamber.
• The patient breathes more easily.
• Auscultation reveals normal, soft, swishing vesicular breath sounds over both lungs.
• The chest X-ray shows a reexpanded lung.

After confirming that the patient no longer needs the chest tube, expect to clamp it for 24 hours. During that time, watch for signs of respiratory distress, which indicate remaining or reaccumulating air. If no signs appear, the doctor will remove the chest tube.

Assisting with chest tube removal

To assist with tube removal, first gather the following equipment: a suture removal kit with forceps and scissors, linen saver pad, sterile petrolatum gauze, several sterile 4″ × 4″ gauze pads, wide adhesive or nonallergenic tape, waterproof trash bag, clean gloves to remove the dressings, and sterile gloves to remove the tube. After you've gathered the necessary equipment, follow these steps:

• If ordered, administer an analgesic about 30 minutes before the procedure to decrease discomfort.

• Place the patient in semi-Fowler's position or on his unaffected side. Place a linen saver pad under the patient's affected side to protect the bed linen from drainage and to provide a place to put the chest tube after removal.

• Put on clean gloves and remove the chest tube dressing with forceps, being careful not to dislodge the chest tube. Discard the soiled dressings in the trash bag.

• After the dressing is removed, the doctor will put on the sterile gloves and cut the anchoring suture. Instruct the patient to exhale and hold his breath or to inhale fully and hold his breath while the doctor quickly pulls out the tube. (Holding his breath will prevent the patient from sucking air into the pleural

space during tube removal.)

• The doctor will place an airtight dressing over the site, taping it securely. Arrange for a portable chest X-ray to confirm that no air has entered the pleural space and that the lung remains expanded.

• Properly dispose of the tube and all soiled equipment.

Monitoring and aftercare

After the chest tube has been removed, assess the patient frequently and check the dressing site for an air leak. Watch for signs of a recurring pneumothorax, subcutaneous emphysema, or infection. Pneumothorax may result from an ineffective seal at the insertion site or from the underlying disease. Subcutaneous emphysema is indicated by a crackling sound heard when the area around the wound is palpated and may also result from a poor seal at the insertion site.

Suggested readings

Butler, S. "Current Trends in Autologous Transfusion," *RN* 52(11):44-55, November 1989.

Erickson, R.S. "Mastering the Ins and Outs of Chest Drainage, Part I," *Nursing89* 19(5):36-43, May 1989.

Erickson, R.S. "Mastering the Ins and Outs of Chest Drainage, Part II," *Nursing89* 19(6):46-49, June 1989.

Kinney, M.R., et al. *AACN's Clinical Reference for Critical-Care Nursing,* 2nd ed. New York: McGraw-Hill Book Co., 1988.

SELF-TEST

Test your respiratory therapy knowledge and skills at your own pace by answering the multiple-choice questions on pages 192 to 195. Answers appear on page 195.

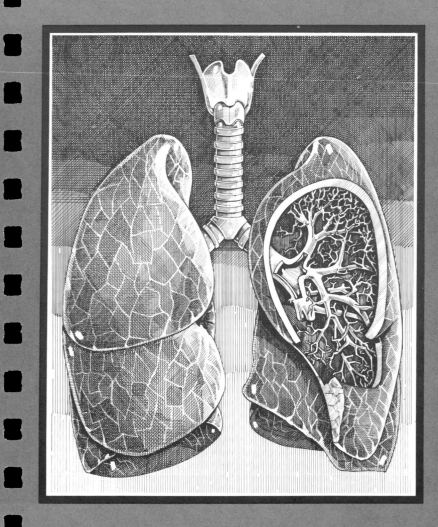

QUESTIONS

1. *Which of the following is not a potential hazard of oxygen therapy?*
a. atelectasis
b. oxygen toxicity
c. increased $PaCO_2$
d. circulatory depression

2. *What's an appropriate oxygen delivery system for a patient with chronic obstructive pulmonary disease (COPD)?*
a. nasal cannula set at a higher flow rate
b. nonrebreather mask
c. partial rebreather mask
d. Venturi mask

3. *What makes this delivery system more appropriate for the COPD patient?*
a. It's a low-flow system.
b. It delivers oxygen accurately to within 1%.
c. It doesn't require humidity.
d. It doesn't confine the patient, so compliance is good.

4. *All of the following may indicate that a patient needs oxygen except:*
a. decreased PaO_2.
b. decreased cardiac output, as with congestive heart failure.
c. increased oxygen demand, as with fever.
d. hemoglobin saturation of 95%.

5. *The patient receiving oxygen through a face mask is at risk for:*
a. aspiration.
b. oxygen toxicity.
c. pressure irritation.
d. all of the above.

6. *After you set up a face mask with a reservoir bag, you should check the bag frequently for:*
a. twisting and kinking.
b. slight deflation on inspiration.
c. condensation collection (if you're using humidified oxygen).
d. all of the above.

7. *If you hear a high-pitched whistling sound after you set up a nasal cannula, suspect that:*

a. the humidifier reservoir is too low.
b. the tubing is pinched.
c. the patient has a nasal obstruction.
d. the high-pressure release valve is malfunctioning.

8. *You'd do all of the following for a child in a croup tent except:*
a. have him sit up or sit in an infant seat.
b. frequently open the croup tent to maintain contact with the child.
c. monitor the temperature of both the child and the croup tent.
d. keep the mattress dry with a rubber sheet.

9. *What precaution prevents aspiration when a patient receives continuous positive airway pressure (CPAP) with a mask?*
a. being NPO for 24 hours
b. receiving prophylactic antibiotics
c. having gastric decompression
d. receiving tube feedings

10. *When you have a patient whose chest tube is being drained by gravity, remember to:*
a. position him on his back.
b. restrict him to bed.
c. make sure the tube is long enough to reach the suction source.
d. keep the collection chamber below chest level.

11. *Stripping a chest tube causes dangerous transient suction that can reach a water pressure of:*
a. -20 cm H_2O.
b. -100 cm H_2O.
c. -300 cm H_2O.
d. -400 cm H_2O.

12. *If you note your patient's chest drainage diminishing to little or nothing after surgery and the water-seal solution creeping higher in the chamber, suspect:*
a. an occluded tube.
b. insufficient suction.
c. an evaporated water seal.
d. a reexpanded lung.

13. *What conclusively indicates lung re-expansion after pleural drainage?*
a. no bubbling in the water-seal chamber
b. a chest X-ray
c. vesicular breath sounds over the peripheral lung areas
d. no fluctuations in the water-seal chamber

14. *Initially, how often should you assess a patient after the doctor has removed his chest tube?*
a. every 5 minutes
b. every 15 minutes for the first hour
c. every hour for the first 8 hours
d. at the change of each shift

15. *How does a water seal create a one-way closed drainage system?*
a. It seals off the tubing from the atmosphere.
b. It lets air bubble out of the pleural space.
c. It lets the patient force air out of the pleural space by coughing or exhaling.
d. It creates a slightly positive pressure in the pleural space.

16. *If a patient's coughing or exhaling causes bubbling in the water-seal chamber, then:*
a. a leak has developed, probably at a tubing connection.
b. the patient still has an air leak in the pleural space.
c. the suction is sufficient.
d. the suction needs to be increased.

17. *For chest drainage of an adult:*
a. you need high negative pressure.
b. the suction level is determined by the patient's condition and the type of drainage.
c. the suction level is determined by its effect on the body tissue in the area that's draining.
d. you need a low negative pressure (between -15 and -20 cm H_2O).

18. *A flutter valve without a water seal:*
a. can be used only for liquid drainage.
b. can be used only for air drainage.
c. won't prevent air from entering the pleural space.
d. won't provide information about air leaks or intrapleural pressure.

19. *Aspirated particles fall into the right bronchus rather than the left because:*
a. the right is a more direct passageway to the trachea.
b. the right is shorter than the left.
c. the right is wider than the left.
d. all of the above.

20. *Which of the following statements is true of surfactant?*
a. It's produced by Type II cells.
b. It prevents total alveolar collapse.
c. It helps air exchange by decreasing surface tension.
d. All of the above.

21. *Oxygenated blood is pumped from the:*
a. lungs to the left atrium via the pulmonary veins.
b. right atrium to the pulmonary veins.
c. left ventricle to the pulmonary arteries.
d. right ventricle to the pulmonary arteries.

22. *In the COPD patient, you'd expect to find:*
a. expiration as much as four times longer than inspiration.
b. inspiration longer than expiration.
c. expiration twice as long as inspiration.
d. expiration equal to inspiration.

23. *What does central cyanosis indicate?*
a. deoxygenated hemoglobin or hypoxia
b. left-to-right cardiac shunting
c. vasoconstriction or diminished blood flow
d. early cardiogenic shock

24. *What complication would you* not *associate with CPAP?*
a. aspiration
b. decreased cardiac output
c. hypoventilation
d. hypervolemia

25. *Respiratory excursion helps you assess:*
a. vibrations.
b. voice sounds.
c. breath sounds.
d. chest movements.

26. *Peripheral cyanosis does* not *affect the:*
a. ears.
b. nail beds.
c. mucous membranes.
d. fingers.

27. *What type of mechanical ventilation synchronizes machine-delivered and patient breaths?*
a. synchronized intermittent mandatory ventilation
b. intermittent mandatory ventilation
c. assist control ventilation
d. positive end-expiratory pressure (PEEP)

28. *Decreased cardiac output, a complication of PEEP, results from:*
a. high intrathoracic pressure.
b. inaccurate machine settings.
c. low intrathoracic pressure.
d. all of the above.

29. *Your assessment of a patient on mechanical ventilation should include:*
a. vital signs.
b. breath sounds.
c. a complete body system review.
d. a neurologic check.

30. *In a patient on PEEP or CPAP, a sudden blood pressure drop, an increased heart rate, decreased urine output, or altered neurologic status points to:*
a. hyperventilation.
b. hypervolemia.
c. hypoventilation.
d. hypovolemia.

31. *In a patient who has undergone bronchoscopy, subcutaneous crepitus may indicate:*
a. tracheal or bronchial perforation.
b. a normal recovery.
c. bronchospasm.
d. infection.

32. *If you don't hear bilateral breath sounds after an oral endotracheal tube has been inserted, suspect that the tube:*
a. is too small for the patient.
b. is in place and breath sounds will start any moment.
c. wasn't inserted far enough.
d. may lie in a mainstem bronchus.

33. *What shouldn't you do during endotracheal extubation?*
a. hyperinflate the patient's lungs with a hand-held resuscitation bag
b. elevate his bed 90 degrees and suction secretions
c. check for air leaks in and around the cuff
d. cut the pilot balloon to deflate it

34. *You probably won't see complications more than 48 hours after a tracheostomy tube insertion.*
a. true
b. false

35. *Incentive spirometry does all of the following* except:
a. increase the effort needed to expand the lung.
b. let you evaluate the effectiveness of deep breathing.
c. replace natural sighing.
d. encourage shallow breathing.

36. *What's usually the most effective sequence for postural drainage?*
a. middle lobe, upper lobe, lower lobe
b. upper lobe, lower lobe, middle lobe
c. lower lobe, middle lobe, upper lobe

37. *You would* not *expect to see a nasopharyngeal airway used in a patient with:*
a. sepsis.
b. a predisposition to nosebleeds.
c. a hemorrhagic disorder.
d. all of the above.

38. *Which symptoms most often point to respiratory dysfunction?*
a. coughing and sputum production
b. dyspnea
c. chest pain
d. all of the above

39. *What's the normal inspiratory-expiratory ratio?*
a. 1:2
b. 2:1
c. 1:1
d. 2:2

40. *In a patient with dark brown or black skin, where would you look for signs of cyanosis?*
a. lips
b. mucous membranes
c. nail beds
d. earlobes

ANSWERS

1. d	**6.** d	**11.** d	**16.** c	**21.** a	**26.** a	**31.** a	**36.** c
2. d	**7.** b	**12.** d	**17.** d	**22.** a	**27.** a	**32.** d	**37.** d
3. b	**8.** b	**13.** b	**18.** d	**23.** a	**28.** a	**33.** d	**38.** d
4. d	**9.** c	**14.** a	**19.** d	**24.** d	**29.** c	**34.** b	**39.** a
5. d	**10.** d	**15.** a	**20.** d	**25.** d	**30.** d	**35.** d	**40.** b

INDEX

INDEX

i refers to an illustration; *t* refers to a table

i refers to an illustration; *t* refers to a table

i refers to an illustration; *t* refers to a table